Walking Western New York With Ryan Young

Walking Western New York
By Ryan Young

© 2025 Ryan Young

All rights reserved.

No part of this publication may be reproduced, stored in a retrieval system, or transmitted in any form or by any means—electronic, mechanical, photocopying, recording, or otherwise—without the prior written permission of the publisher, except in the case of brief quotations used in critical articles or reviews.

This book is a work of nonfiction. While every effort has been made to ensure accuracy, the author and publisher assume no responsibility for errors or omissions, or for the use or interpretation of the information contained herein.

ISBN: 978-1-945423-71-0

Published by:
5 Stones Publishing
info@ILNcenter.com

Printed in the United States of America.

For information about this and other titles from 5 Stones Publishing, please contact the publisher or visit www.ilncenter.com

Introduction

At 5, my life took an unexpected turn. A car accident left me with a traumatic brain injury, and doctors questioned whether I'd ever walk again. The journey to recovery was long and challenging, requiring me to relearn basic functions like walking and talking. Through determination, faith, and the unwavering support of my family, I not only regained these abilities but also discovered a renewed purpose in life.

Today, I hold a third-degree black belt in Karate, have completed a marathon, and continue to embrace life's adventures. One of my most fulfilling experiences was traveling to the Andes Mountains in Peru, where I assisted in constructing a school for the deaf. These experiences have deepened my commitment to helping others lead healthy and fulfilling lives.

As an inspirational speaker, my mission is to encourage people to "get moving"—physically, mentally, and spiritually. In this book, I share my love for the outdoors and offer suggestions for places to explore, regardless of your physical abilities. Life is a gift, and I believe everyone deserves the opportunity to experience its wonders to the fullest.

Contents

Letchworth State Park 7

Old Man River 13

Fort Niagara 17

Watkins Glen 21

Stony Brook 25

Rock City 29

Green Lakes State Park 35

Destiny USA Mall 37

Fillmore Glen State Park 43

Jamestown Comedy Central Park 47

Powder Mills Park 51

Eastview Mall 55

Whirlpool State Park 59

Rochester Square 63

Ellison Park 67

Finger Lakes National Forest 71

Green Park 79

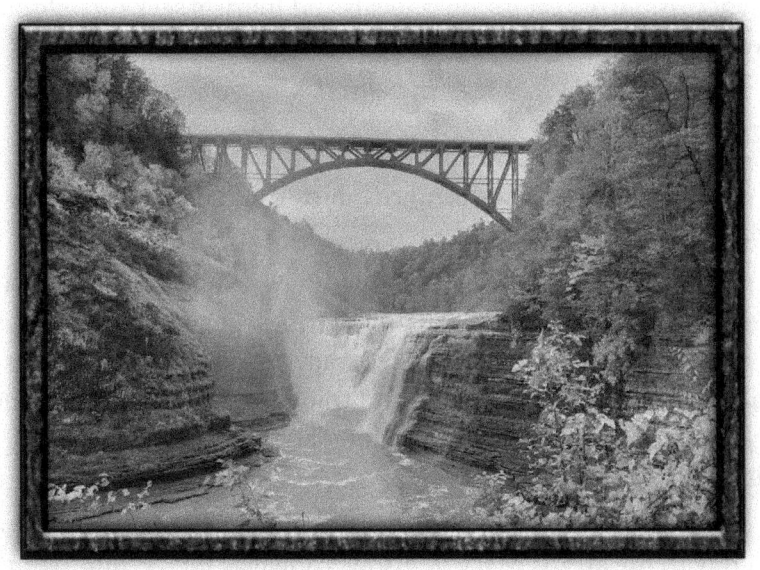

Letchworth State Park

Location

Letchworth State Park is nestled in the scenic region of Western New York, which is part of the larger Finger Lakes area. This park is located in Livingston and Wyoming counties, about 35 miles southwest of Rochester and 60 miles southeast of Buffalo. The region is known for its picturesque landscapes, featuring rolling hills, lush forests, and numerous lakes and rivers. Western New York is characterized by its rural charm contrasted with nearby urban centers, offering a blend of cultural attractions and natural beauty. The Genesee River, which runs through Letchworth State Park, contributes significantly to the area's scenic allure, cutting a deep gorge through the park that has earned it the nickname "Grand Canyon of the East."

This part of New York is also famous for its vibrant fall foliage, making autumn a particularly spectacular time to visit. The area's climate is influenced by the Great Lakes, leading to cold, snowy winters and warm, humid summers. Letchworth's location makes it an accessible retreat for both locals and tourists seeking outdoor adventures amidst stunning natural settings.

History

Letchworth State Park has a rich historical tapestry that adds depth to its natural beauty.

Native American Presence: Before European settlers, the area was home to several Native American tribes, including the Seneca Nation, part of the Iroquois Confederacy. The Genesee River was vital for fishing, transportation, and trade. Archaeological evidence suggests human activity in the region dating back thousands of years.

Mary Jemison: One of the most famous historical figures associated with the area is Mary Jemison, known as the "White Woman of the Genesee." Captured by the Seneca in the 1750s, she chose to live with them and her story is part of the park's lore, with her grave located within the park.

William Pryor Letchworth: The park's modern history begins with William Pryor Letchworth, who in the mid to late 19th century, bought land along the Genesee River to preserve its natural beauty. He developed the area into a private park, opening it to the public in 1906. After his death in 1910, he bequeathed the land to New York State with the stipulation it be used as a public park.

State Park Designation: In 1907, before Letchworth's death, the state had already started discussions on turning it into a state park. It officially became Letchworth State Park in 1907, one of the first state parks in the United States, showcasing progressive conservation efforts of the time.

Development and Conservation: Over the 20th century, the park saw various developments like the building of trails, picnic areas, and the Glen Iris Inn, originally Letchworth's home, now a hotel. Conservation efforts have included restoring natural habitats and managing the impact of tourism on the environment.

Cultural and Historical Preservation: The park contains several historical structures, including the William Pryor Letchworth

Museum, which educates visitors on the history of the park and its significance. There are also remnants of Seneca culture and the industrial history of the area, like old railroad grades now turned into hiking trails.

Modern Challenges: Today, the park faces challenges like erosion control due to its unique geological features and managing visitor impact to preserve its natural and historical integrity.

This history not only shapes the physical landscape of Letchworth but also enriches the visitor experience, offering a glimpse into the layers of human interaction with this remarkable natural space.

Terrain

Hiking in Letchworth State Park offers a diverse range of terrains that cater to both novice and experienced hikers. The park encompasses over 14,000 acres, with the Genesee River carving out a dramatic gorge that defines much of the landscape. Here's what hikers can expect:

Gorges and Cliffs: The park is famous for its deep gorges, with cliffs rising up to 600 feet, providing breathtaking views but also necessitating caution. Trails often run along the edge of these cliffs, offering scenic overlooks but requiring careful navigation.

Forest Trails: Much of the park is covered by dense, deciduous forests. Trails weave through these woodlands, providing shade and a habitat for various wildlife. The forest floor can be uneven with roots and rocks, which adds to the hiking challenge.

River Access: Several trails lead down to the Genesee River, where the terrain becomes more rugged, with rocky riverbanks and sometimes slippery conditions due to water proximity. There are flat areas by the river that are perfect for picnicking or fishing but require careful descent and ascent.

Historical Paths: Some trails follow old railroad beds, which are relatively flat and wide, offering easier hiking paths. However, even these paths can include sections with steeper inclines or declines as they traverse the varied topography of the park.

Elevation Changes: Hikers should prepare for significant elevation gains and losses, particularly when exploring the different levels of the gorge. Trails like the Gorge Trail involve numerous stairs and steep sections, making them more strenuous.

Seasonal Variations: The terrain can change with the seasons. In winter, trails might be covered with snow and ice, making them more treacherous, while in spring or after rain, mud can make certain paths slippery.

Hiking in Letchworth requires good footwear, an awareness of one's physical limits, and an appreciation for the natural beauty that comes with navigating such varied landscapes.

Ryan's Notes:

This was mine and Jamie's first adventure together with many more to come. We went through many different paths somewhere more flat than others, we went towards the water which was a beach with small and large rocks. This is where Jamie took a picture of me. We then proceeded to a trail that was hilly. I walked past Jamie and walked up the hill with no problem, however Jamie had an issue and called me back. So I came back and helped her up the hill. So we got up the hill and continued our walk. We enjoyed the beauty and the nature that is at Letchworth Park. We saw the log cabin to use if you choose to stay overnight. We also saw the three different falls in Letchworth as well; these falls are called upper, middle and lower falls. We ended up leaving due to rain.

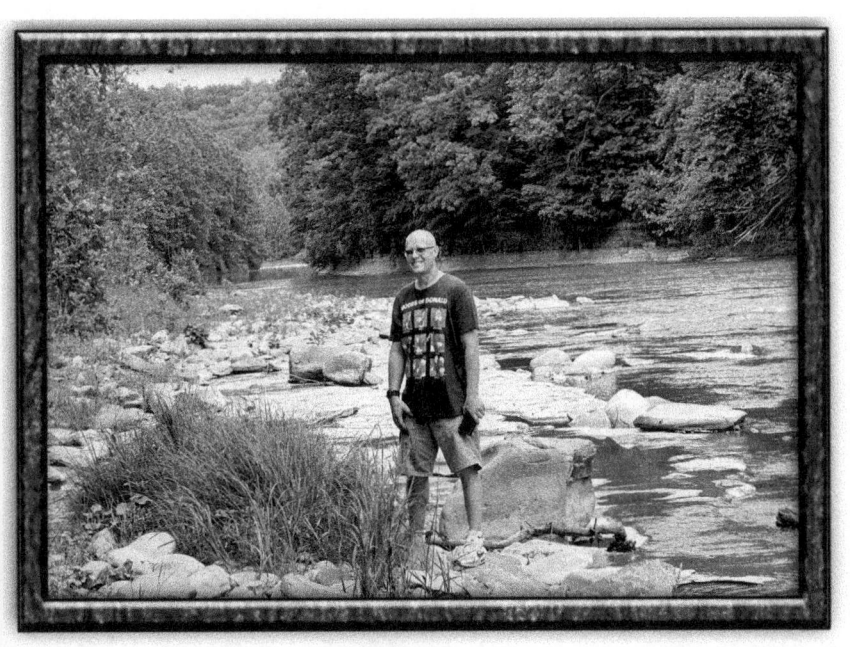

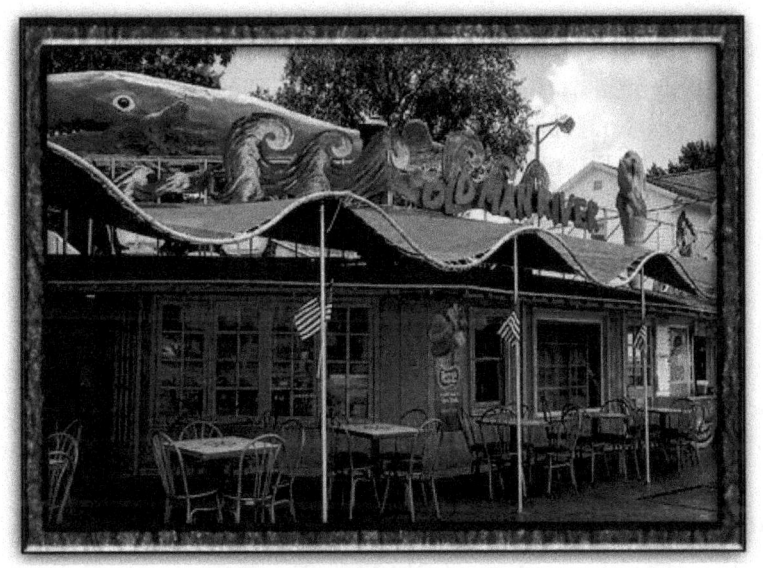

Old Man River

Location

Old Man River is not an actual river but refers to a well-known seasonal restaurant and entertainment venue located in Tonawanda, New York. Tonawanda is a town in Erie County, part of Western New York, situated along the Niagara River.

This location places it directly across from Niawanda Park, offering a scenic view of the Niagara River, which is one of the defining features of the region. Tonawanda is just north of Buffalo, providing easy access for both locals and tourists from the surrounding areas, including Southern Ontario, Canada. The proximity to the Niagara River makes this spot a popular destination for those looking to enjoy outdoor dining with river views, especially during the summer months when the restaurant is open.

History

Old Man River's story begins in the 1970s when Dick Bratek saw the potential in the scenic banks of the Niagara River. He opened a seasonal eatery that would soon become a beloved fixture in Tonawanda. From humble beginnings, Old Man River has grown into a local institution known for its seafood, especially the clams, and its relaxed, outdoor dining atmosphere.a

Over the decades, the restaurant has seen different owners, each adding their unique touch to the establishment. Whether it was expanding the menu, introducing live music, or enhancing the riverside deck for better views, the essence of enjoying a meal by the river has remained unchanged. This continuity has made Old Man River more than just a restaurant; it's a cultural landmark where countless memories have been made.

The seasonal operation of Old Man River, opening from late spring to early fall, reflects the rhythm of life in Western New York, where summer is celebrated with outdoor activities before the onset of winter. This seasonality adds to the venue's charm, making it a symbol of summer along the Niagara River.

Despite facing its share of challenges, including economic fluctuations and shifts in local regulations, Old Man River has shown resilience. Its continued popularity is a testament to the community's affection for this unique spot. The restaurant has become woven into the social fabric of Tonawanda, often playing host to local festivals and community events, contributing significantly to the cultural life of the area.

Old Man River isn't just a place to eat; it's a piece of local history and identity, embodying the spirit of Tonawanda's riverside community life.

Terrain

Old Man River is situated along the banks of the Niagara River, which forms part of the border between the United States and Canada. The area around Tonawanda and this stretch of the river is characterized by its natural beauty, offering a blend of urban and natural landscapes:

The terrain around this part of the Niagara River is relatively flat compared to more rugged hiking areas, making it accessible for a variety of outdoor activities. Here's what you might expect if you explore the surrounding area on foot:

Riverfront Trails: There are several walking and biking paths that run parallel to the river, like the Niawanda Park Trail. These trails provide easy, level walking with panoramic views of the Niagara River. The paths are often paved or well-maintained gravel, suitable for all ages and fitness levels.

Parks and Green Spaces: Niawanda Park, directly across from Old Man River, offers grassy areas, picnic spots, and playgrounds. The park is a gentle introduction to outdoor activities with a focus more on relaxation than on rugged hiking. However, it's an excellent place to start a leisurely walk or run.

Waterfront Access: The riverbank itself can be muddy or rocky in places, and while not typically considered "hiking," exploring closer to the water's edge might involve navigating through small, natural obstacles like driftwood or rocks. This part of the river is calm, making it ideal for fishing or bird watching rather than for challenging treks.

Urban Interface: Hiking here means you're never far from urban amenities. You might walk from riverside paths directly into the neighborhoods of Tonawanda or North Tonawanda, where the terrain shifts from natural to man-made with sidewalks and streets.

Seasonal Variations: In winter, these paths might be under snow or ice, changing the hiking experience to one that requires more caution and perhaps even snowshoes for deeper snow. Spring and fall bring out the best in the area's natural beauty with blooming or falling leaves, while summer is prime for water-based activities.

Views and Wildlife: The riverside trails offer views of passing boats, the distant skyline of Niagara Falls, and sometimes wildlife like waterfowl, making for a serene hiking experience. The area is known for its birdwatching opportunities, particularly during migration seasons.

This part of Western New York combines the tranquility of river life with the convenience of urban accessibility, making it a unique place for those who prefer a more relaxed, scenic walk over a strenuous hike.

Ryan's Notes:

When Jamie and I would get back from the state parks I would go to 9 round boxing then go to old man river to join my friends from slow spokes to do a 10 mile bike ride through the Tonawanda area. Here we would grab dinner and listen to whatever band was playing. Sometimes, especially when they played rock and roll, I would dance. During the Fourth of July we saw Aerial dancers which was fun to watch after my bike ride. We also saw the fireworks across the river that night as well.

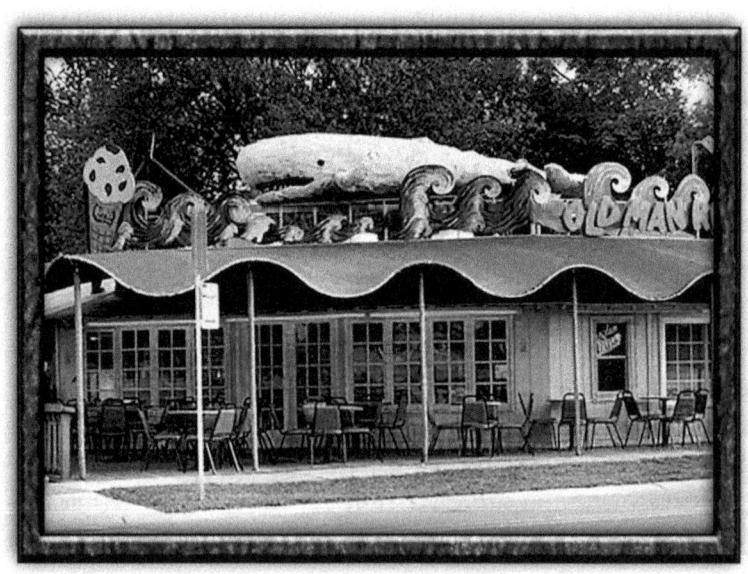

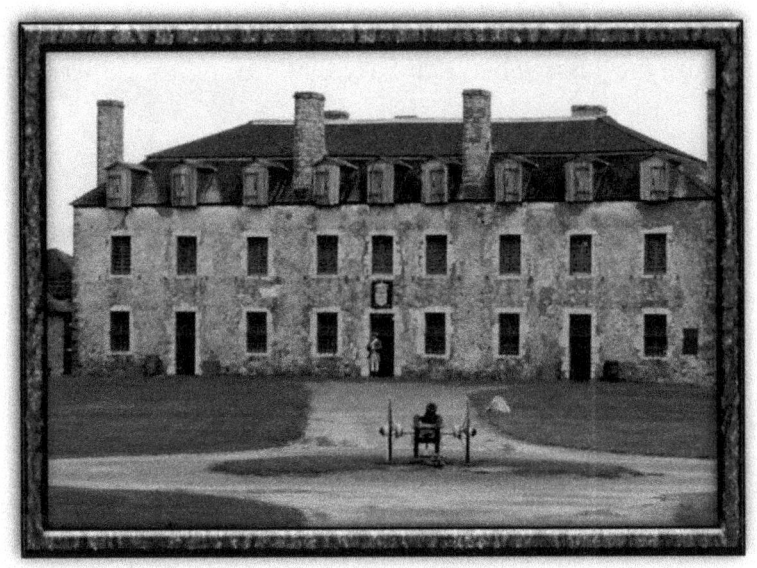

Fort Niagara

Location

Fort Niagara is located at the mouth of the Niagara River, where it flows into Lake Ontario, in the town of Youngstown, New York.

This strategic location places Fort Niagara at a pivotal point between two important bodies of water, making it historically significant for both military and trade purposes. Youngstown is in Niagara County, roughly 20 miles north of Buffalo and just south of the border with Canada. The fort overlooks the river and lake, offering panoramic views and a commanding presence at one of the Great Lakes' most critical passages. This location not only adds to the fort's historical importance but also its scenic appeal for visitors today.

History

Fort Niagara's history is as layered and complex as the strategic landscape it oversees. Initially, the area was significant for the Seneca Nation, who utilized its position at the mouth of the Niagara River for fishing and trade. The French, recognizing its strategic value, established the first fort in 1726 to control the fur trade and secure the passage between Lake Ontario and the upper Great Lakes.

This fort became a focal point during the French and Indian War, changing hands in 1759 when the British captured it, ushering in a new era of British control until the American Revolution. The fort's strategic importance made it a pivotal point in colonial conflicts, witnessing the Siege of Fort Niagara in 1759, which was one of the war's decisive engagements.

During the American Revolution, Fort Niagara remained under British control until it was officially handed over to the United States in 1796 as part of Jay's Treaty. However, the War of 1812 saw the British briefly reoccupy the fort before returning it to American hands at the conflict's conclusion.

The 19th century saw Fort Niagara transition from a purely military outpost to an educational institution, hosting the U.S. Army's School of Application for Infantry and Cavalry, which later moved to Fort Leavenworth. In the 20th century, through both World Wars, the fort served various military functions, including as a training center.

After World War II, with the fort's military relevance diminishing, New York State took over much of it in 1963 to preserve its historical structures as a state park. Now managed by the New York State Office of Parks, Recreation, and Historic Preservation, Fort Niagara stands as a testament to centuries of military, cultural, and diplomatic history. Visitors today can delve into this rich tapestry through guided tours, living history programs, and exhibits that explore the interactions between French, British, and American influences, alongside the enduring presence of the Seneca Nation.

The fort's story is not merely one of battles and treaties; it's also a narrative of cultural exchange, the evolution of military strategy, and the enduring significance of this strategic point on the Great Lakes.

Terrain

When visiting Fort Niagara, the terrain around this historic site offers a blend of historical structures, natural landscapes, and waterfront access:

Upon entering the fort, visitors will encounter a mix of flat, well-maintained paths and cobblestone or brick surfaces typical of historic military installations. The fort itself is built on relatively level ground, with various buildings, bastions, and defensive structures to explore. The paths within the fort are designed for ease of access, allowing visitors of all ages to navigate through history with comfort.Outside the fort's immediate structures, the terrain diversifies:

Riverside and Lakefront: To the north, the Niagara River meets Lake Ontario, providing expansive views and access to the water's edge. Here, the ground can be grassy or sandy, with some areas featuring rocky outcrops. The shoreline is generally gentle, suitable for picnicking or fishing, but caution is advised near the water, especially during high winds or wave conditions.

Parkland and Green Spaces: The state park surrounding Fort Niagara includes well-manicured lawns, picnic areas, and playgrounds. These areas are mostly flat, ideal for leisurely walks or family outings. The park also maintains several trails that offer easy walks with historical markers and scenic overlooks of the river and lake.

Historical Reenactment Areas: In parts used for living history demonstrations, the terrain might include setups mimicking past military camps or settlements, where the ground could be less uniform, featuring dirt or gravel surfaces to reflect historical authenticity.

Seasonal Changes: In winter, the area can be covered with snow, altering the hiking experience. Trails might be icy, requiring appropriate footwear. Conversely, spring and fall bring vibrant colors to the landscape, with autumn particularly noted for its spectacular foliage around the fort.

Accessibility: The fort and its surrounding park areas are generally accessible for those with mobility aids, thanks to paved or hard-packed paths. However, some historical areas of the fort or less-traveled paths might present challenges due to uneven ground or steps.

Overall, the terrain at Fort Niagara is diverse enough to offer both a historical journey through time and a pleasant outdoor experience. Whether you're exploring the fort's ancient walls, walking along the river, or enjoying the park's recreational facilities, the site provides a varied landscape that complements its rich history.

Ryan's Notes:

We drove to the Old Fort Niagara and parked by the beach area. We went down the hill onto the beach, walked across the beach toward the large boulder which I walked onto, making Jamie nervous. Once I got off the boulders we walked all the way back on the beach I helped Jamie up a huge hill and back onto the pavement. We saw different buildings at the park then went past the marinia to watch the sailboats in the water in lake Ontarino. We left the park and continued into the town and kept on walking. Eventually we turned around and went to a dinner in town to have lunch. After lunch we went back to the car and headed back home because the day was cloudy and it started to rain.

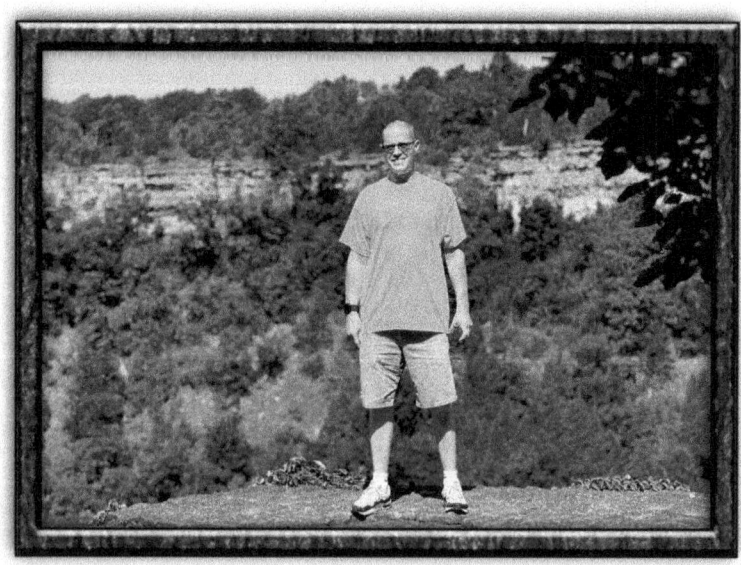

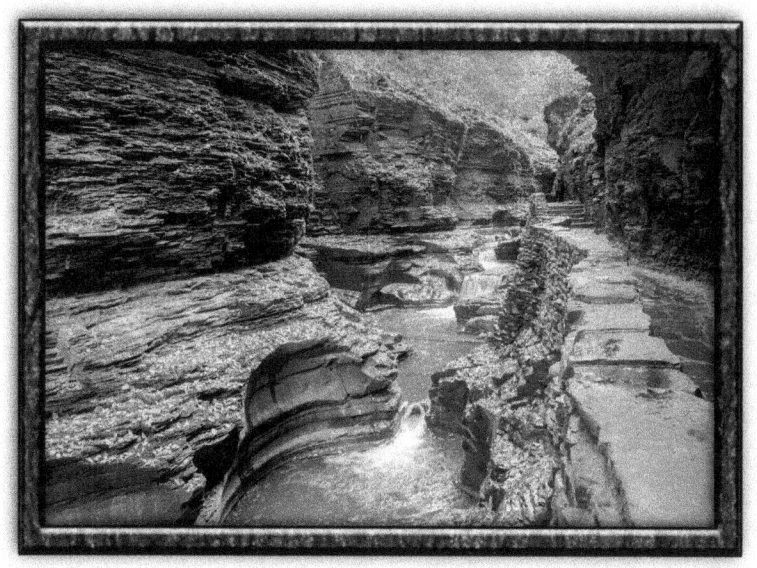

Watkins Glen

Location

Watkins Glen is located in the heart of the Finger Lakes region, specifically in Schuyler County, New York. Situated at the southern tip of Seneca Lake, which is the largest of the Finger Lakes, Watkins Glen is in the village of the same name.

Watkins Glen is approximately 250 miles northwest of New York City, 60 miles southwest of Syracuse, and 30 miles west of Ithaca. This positioning makes it part of Western New York, although it's often considered more central within the state due to its placement in the Finger Lakes area. The village lies between the towns of Dix and Reading, with Watkins Glen State Park almost within walking distance from the village center, providing easy access to its natural attractions. The area is known for its scenic beauty, with the surrounding hills, vineyards, and the deep, clear waters of Seneca Lake defining the landscape.

History

The history of Watkins Glen is as intricate and fascinating as the gorge that runs through it. Originally, the area was home to the Seneca tribe of the Iroquois Confederacy, who made use of the land's natural resources for sustenance and trade. The village's name honors Dr. Samuel Watkins, who in the early 19th century, spearheaded development by establishing mills along the gorge's waterways.

In the 1800s, Watkins Glen became an industrial center, particularly after the railroad connected the village in 1871, facilitating the growth of mills, factories, and a salt industry thanks to local saline springs. However, the true character of Watkins Glen was shaped by its stunning natural beauty. The gorge, with its cascading waterfalls and winding trails, became a draw for tourists. By 1863, community leaders purchased the land for public enjoyment, and in 1924, Watkins Glen State Park was formally established, marking it as one of New York's earliest state parks.

The modern identity of Watkins Glen is also tied to its racing heritage. The first road races in the village occurred in 1948, leading to the opening of the Watkins Glen International racetrack in 1956, which has since become a mecca for motorsport fans, hosting prestigious events like the Formula One U.S. Grand Prix and NASCAR races.

Beyond its natural and racing allure, Watkins Glen has a rich cultural history. It famously hosted the Summer Jam at Watkins Glen in 1973, one of the largest rock concerts ever, and has become a focal point for wine tourism due to its location near the vineyards of Seneca Lake.

Throughout its history, there has been a concerted effort to preserve the natural beauty of Watkins Glen while accommodating human activity. The park's development includes pathways, bridges, and stairs designed to provide access while protecting the environment. This balance reflects Watkins Glen's journey from a Native American settlement, through industrial growth, to becoming a cherished destination for both its natural wonders and cultural events.

Terrain

Visitors to Watkins Glen can expect a diverse and captivating terrain, both within the village and at the state park:

The most iconic feature of Watkins Glen is undoubtedly its state park, which centers around a dramatic gorge cut by Glen Creek. Here, the terrain is marked by:

Gorge Trails: The Gorge Trail is the star attraction, featuring nearly 200 stone steps and pathways that weave through the rock formations, under waterfalls, and across stone bridges. The trail is relatively narrow with many inclines and declines, offering breathtaking views but requiring careful navigation, especially when wet or icy.

Waterfalls and Cliffs: Along the trail, visitors will encounter several waterfalls, with the most notable being Rainbow Falls, Cavern Cascade, and the towering Central Cascade. The trail often hugs the edges of cliffs, so protective railings are in place, but caution is still advised.

Natural Surfaces: The paths are a mix of natural stone, gravel, and occasionally paved sections. The uneven, rocky terrain means sturdy footwear is essential, especially where water might make the stones slippery.

Seasonal Changes: In spring and fall, the trails can be lush with foliage or vibrant with autumn colors, respectively. Winter transforms the park into a frosty wonderland, though some areas might be closed due to ice, and special winter access might be limited to safer, less steep paths.

Outside the gorge:

Seneca Lake Shoreline: The lakefront provides a contrast with the rugged gorge, offering flat, grassy, or pebbled areas for picnicking, fishing, or simply enjoying the view. Public docks and boat launches are also available, allowing for water activities.

Overall, Watkins Glen presents a tapestry of terrains from the rugged, nature-infused trails of the state park to the calm, picturesque settings of the village and lake. This variety makes it a destination for both adventure seekers and those looking for serene beauty.

Ryan's Notes:

This was mine and Jamie's first weekend trip. We left on a Friday and came back on Saturday. It was a beautiful sunny day when we got to Watkins Glen. There was a festival going on which made the park full with a lot of people. We parked the car, and started walking before actually getting to the gorge part there is a playground for the kids. So we walked up stairs and more stairs all the way to the top. By then I was a ways ahead and had to wait for Jamie. Once Jamie saw me I kept going. The neat part of Wakitin Glen is the walkways are mostly natural and you can walk and look down to see the rapids and the falls. Every path has stairs or very rough terrain. We walked through the park down the stairs to Burger King for lunch. After lunch we walked around the park to get to the car and headed to find a hotel to spend the night. We actually didn't go directly to the hotel but to another park.

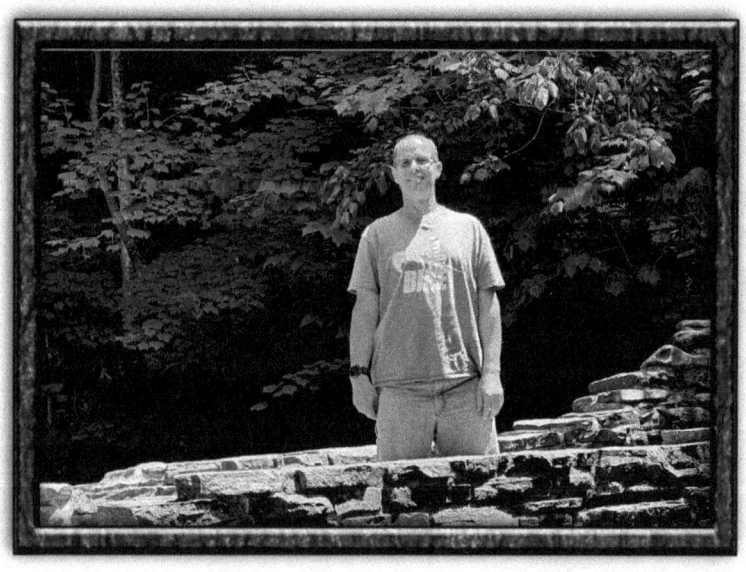

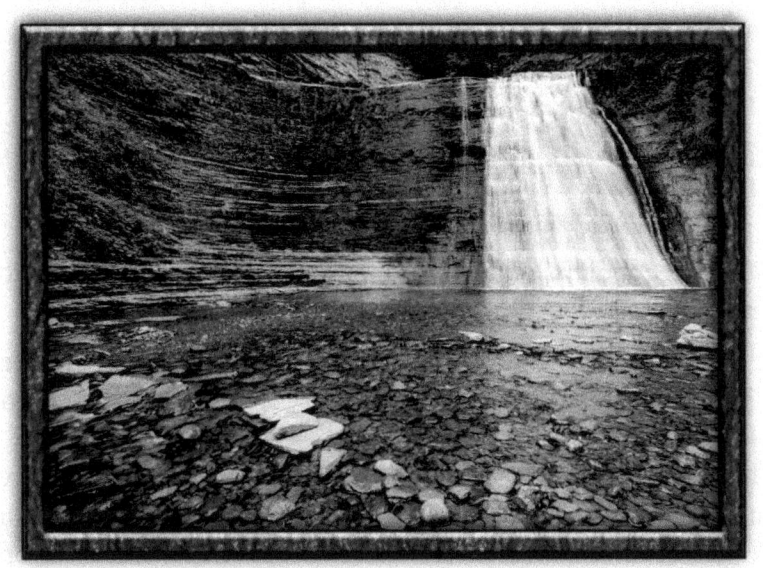

Stony Brook

Location

Stony Brook State Park is found in the rolling hills of Western New York, specifically in Steuben County. It's nestled near the town of Dansville, offering a serene escape not far from urban centers.

The park is approximately 45 miles south of Rochester and about 70 miles east of Buffalo, making it a convenient getaway for those in the greater Rochester or Finger Lakes region. Stony Brook State Park lies in an area known for its scenic beauty, with the park itself cut through by a rugged gorge, providing a stark contrast to the surrounding pastoral landscapes.

History

Stony Brook State Park's history is a narrative of transformation and preservation, reflecting the broader story of land use and conservation in the United States. The area where the park now stands was once a favorite among Native Americans for its natural resources, with evidence suggesting the presence of settlements near what is now the park.

In the late 19th century, after the arrival of the railroad in 1883, the region around Stony Brook became a popular summer destination for those escaping the heat and hustle of urban life. Resorts and summer homes sprang up, capitalizing on the area's natural beauty and the cooling waters of Stony Brook. However, by the 1920s, this popularity waned, and the area saw a decline in resort activities.

New York State saw an opportunity to preserve this scenic area for public enjoyment, and in 1928, it was established as Stony Brook State Park. This move was part of a broader initiative during the early 20th century to create state parks for recreation and conservation. The park was further developed during the Great Depression by works of the Civilian Conservation Corps (CCC) and the Works Progress Administration (WPA). These programs left a lasting legacy in the form of trails, bridges, and park infrastructure, much of which can still be seen today, blending seamlessly with the natural landscape.

The park's history is not just one of leisure but also of stewardship. Efforts have been made to maintain the ecological integrity of the gorge and its waterfall systems while providing access for visitors. Over the years, Stony Brook has evolved from a seasonal retreat for the wealthy to a state park enjoyed by diverse groups seeking to connect with nature. Its history is a testament to how natural beauty, once at risk of being lost to development or neglect, can be preserved for future generations to explore and appreciate.

Terrain

Visitors to Stony Brook State Park will encounter a diverse and engaging terrain that combines natural beauty with a history of conservation efforts:

Gorge and Trails: The centerpiece of the park is the gorge carved by Stony Brook, offering a series of trails that follow the stream, leading visitors through a landscape of cliffs, waterfalls, and dense woodland. The Gorge Trail, in particular, is known for its scenic beauty, featuring numerous steps carved into the rock and bridges that cross the brook. This trail can be steep at times, with uneven, rocky surfaces that require careful footing, especially when wet.

Waterfalls: Along the trail, visitors will encounter several waterfalls, with the most notable being the Lower Falls, which drops into a picturesque pool. The terrain around these falls can be slippery, so caution is advised.

Upper and Lower Park: The upper park is more forested and offers a contrast with wider, less rugged trails suitable for hiking or cross-country skiing in winter. The lower park, where the gorge is, presents a more challenging terrain with its narrow, winding paths and elevation changes.

Riverside and Picnic Areas: Beyond the gorge, the park has flat, grassy areas ideal for picnicking, camping, or simply relaxing by the water. These spaces are less demanding, providing easy access to the brook for fishing or wading.

Seasonal Variations: The terrain changes with the seasons. Spring brings lush greenery and flowing water, summer offers the perfect backdrop for outdoor activities, while autumn transforms the park into a palette of fall colors. Winter blankets the area in snow, altering the hiking experience to one of quiet, serene beauty, though some trails might be closed or require winter footwear.

Historical Structures: The impact of the CCC and WPA is still visible in the form of stone work, bridges, and shelters, adding historical texture to the natural landscape. These structures are often part of the hiking experience, blending human history with the natural terrain.

Overall, Stony Brook State Park offers a mix of rugged adventure and serene exploration. Visitors should come prepared for varied conditions, from the demanding climbs of the gorge to the tranquil walks by the brook, ensuring a memorable experience of Western New York's natural heritage.

Ryan's Notes:

We drove to Stony Brook. There is a pool where the falls circulate it, we couldn't go in because there was no lifeguard. So we started to climb on the path which goes higher and higher. And the pathways get more narrow. There are three different pathways, I went ahead with no problem. I didn't see Jamie fall and some people helped her. They took her to their campsite and tried to call Me. Jamie Asked Me Where Are You? I said just walking in stony brook. Jamie asked me to meet me at the parking lot and he said ok. As I kept walking I found the dirt roads and saw the workers on the four wheeler. Jamie got to the parking lot without me. Jamie got a hold of me. Ask where are you? I said on the dirt roads. So Jamie found the park ranger. The ranger asked her if she had a picture and she said yes. She showed the picture to the ranger and the workers. The workers said yes we saw him would you like for us to pick him up she said yes please. Jamie called me and told me to stay where I'm at so I did and the workers picked me up and I was telling them jokes and laughing. Jamie and the ranger heard me through the walkie telling jokes.

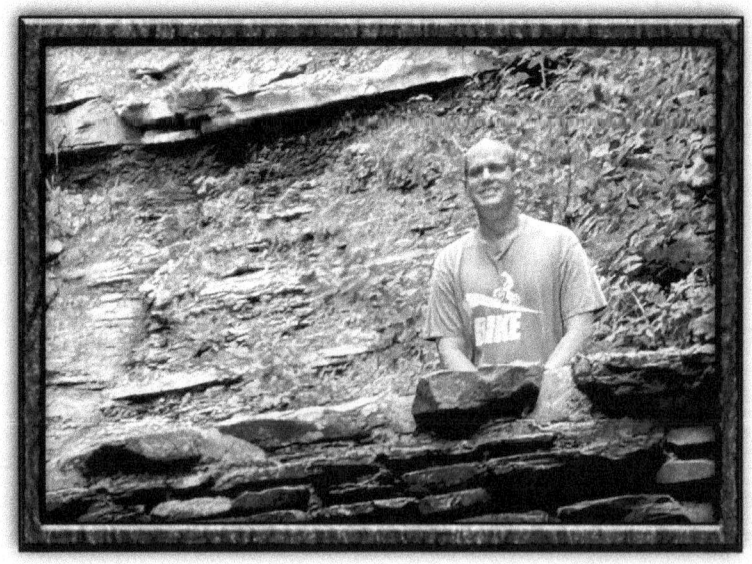

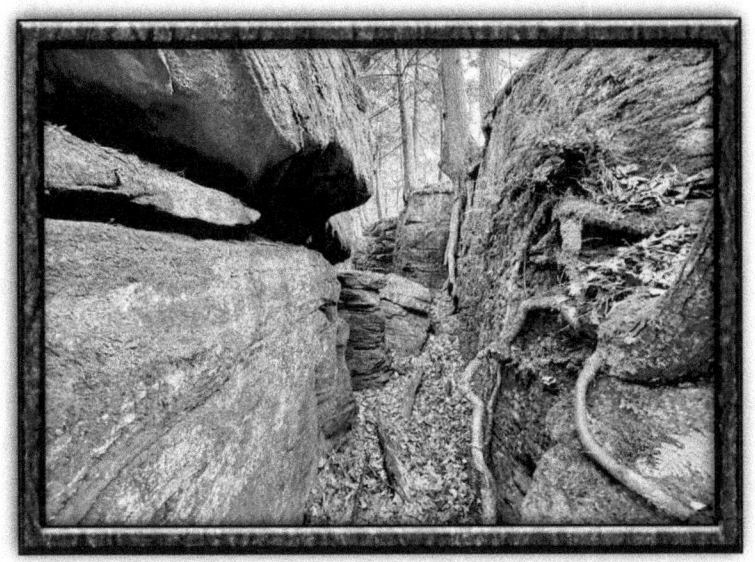

Rock City

Location

Rock City, also known as Little Rock City, is situated within Rock City State Forest, near the city of Salamanca in Cattaraugus County, Western New York.

This unique geological area is just a short drive from Salamanca, which itself is nestled in the Allegheny River valley and part of the Allegany Indian Reservation of the Seneca Nation. Rock City is approximately 70 miles south of Buffalo, making it an accessible natural wonder for those exploring this part of the state. The park is near the border with Pennsylvania, offering a blend of rugged wilderness and local culture in this corner of New York.

History

Rock City's history intertwines with both geological formation and human interaction, offering a narrative that spans millions of years yet is deeply rooted in the more recent past of Western New York:

Geologically, Rock City formed over 320 million years ago during the Mississippian period when layers of sandstone were deposited by ancient seas. Over time, these layers were uplifted and eroded, creating the maze of rock formations we see today. This natural wonder includes towering rock formations, crevices, and overhangs, giving the area its "city-like" appearance.

In terms of human history, the Seneca Nation, part of the Iroquois Confederacy, have lived in the region for centuries, and the area around Rock City would have been known to them. However, there isn't a specific, detailed historical record of their interaction with this exact location, as their presence in the broader area is well-established.

The modern history of Rock City as a public attraction begins in the early 20th century. The site was largely popularized by local residents and tourists seeking out the natural oddities of the region. By the 1920s, Rock City was being promoted as a tourist destination, with pathways and stairs built to make the formations more accessible.

In 1931, the land was acquired by New York State, and Rock City became part of what is now Rock City State Forest. This acquisition ensured the preservation of the site for public enjoyment and study. The Civilian Conservation Corps (CCC) played a significant role during the Great Depression, improving access with trails and steps, many of which visitors still use today.

Over the years, Rock City has evolved from a local curiosity to a recognized geological site, drawing visitors interested in its natural beauty, unique rock formations, and the peaceful forest setting. Educational initiatives have also highlighted the geological significance of the area, making it a point of interest for those studying or simply appreciating natural history.

The history of Rock City is not only about the age of the rocks but also about how this natural wonder has been valued and preserved by generations, providing a place where education, recreation, and natural beauty meet.

Terrain

Visitors to Rock City in Salamanca will encounter a terrain that is both unique and challenging, offering an adventure unlike any other in Western New York:

Rock Formations: The primary feature of Rock City is its labyrinth of massive sandstone boulders, some standing over 30 feet high, creating a maze of narrow passages, archways, and small caves. This creates an otherworldly landscape where visitors can explore through, over, and around these geological wonders. The terrain here is rocky, uneven, and requires careful navigation.

Natural Trails: There are well-worn paths and steps, often made from the same stone, that guide visitors through this natural city. These paths can be steep, with some areas requiring climbing or scrambling over rocks. The trails are not paved but are maintained for safety, though they still offer a rugged hiking experience.

Forest Surroundings: Beyond the rock formations, the area is enveloped by the forest of Rock City State Forest, providing a contrast with softer, more typical woodland terrain. Here, the ground can be covered with leaves, pine needles, or ferns, offering easier walking but with the occasional root or rock to navigate.

Elevation Changes: The layout of Rock City involves significant elevation changes as you move through different parts of the rock maze. There are natural staircases and inclines, which can be quite steep, making for a physically engaging visit.

Seasonal Variations: The terrain's nature changes with the seasons. In spring, mosses and ferns can make rocks slippery, while autumn turns the forest into a colorful backdrop to the grey of the rocks. Winter might bring a layer of snow or ice, adding a level of difficulty and beauty to the exploration, though caution is necessary.

Views and Vistas: While much of the exploration is within the rock formations, there are points where the terrain opens up, offering views through the trees or from atop higher boulders, providing a sense of scale to the area's natural architecture.

Accessibility: Due to the rugged nature of the site, some parts of Rock City might not be easily accessible for those with mobility issues. However, the park does its best to provide some accessible paths around the periphery for a taste of the experience.

Visiting Rock City is like stepping into a natural cathedral of stone, where each turn through the rocks reveals new wonders. It's an adventure that combines the thrill of exploration with the awe of geological time, all within the serene setting of a state forest.

Ryan's Notes:

This was quite the adventure. The terrain is very rocky. It was a bright, sunny and warm day. This place was very easy to get lost in with the huge boulders that look like they come out of the ground from nowhere. We saw old bridges and many small creeks. Some of these boulders actually create their own paths and are so talls. As we kept walking on the path, further and further into the forest, Jamie's phone died so she called me over and asked how far the path goes. I said I don't know, we weren't sure if we were walking in circles. I asked Jamie if she wanted me to get help. So I called the forest ranger, because I'm a neighborhood watcher. As I was on the phone with the ranger a biker passed us Jamie asked if this was the correct path but he didn't answer. The ranger told us they were 40 minutes away. So we kept walking and finally found the paved road. We started walking one way, not sure it was the correct way, it wasn't, until we found a park ranger form Allegany State Park walking her dog and said she would help us find our car. I called the park ranger from Rock city back and told them we found help. We thanked the park ranger from Allegany park and headed home.

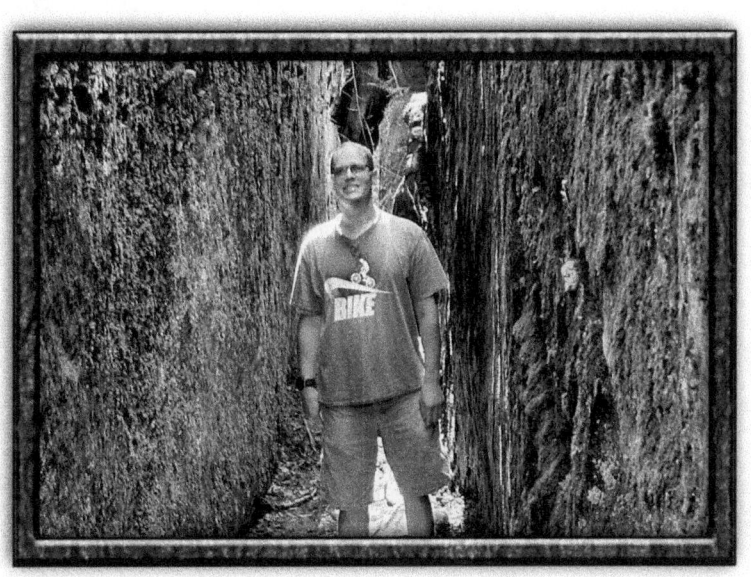

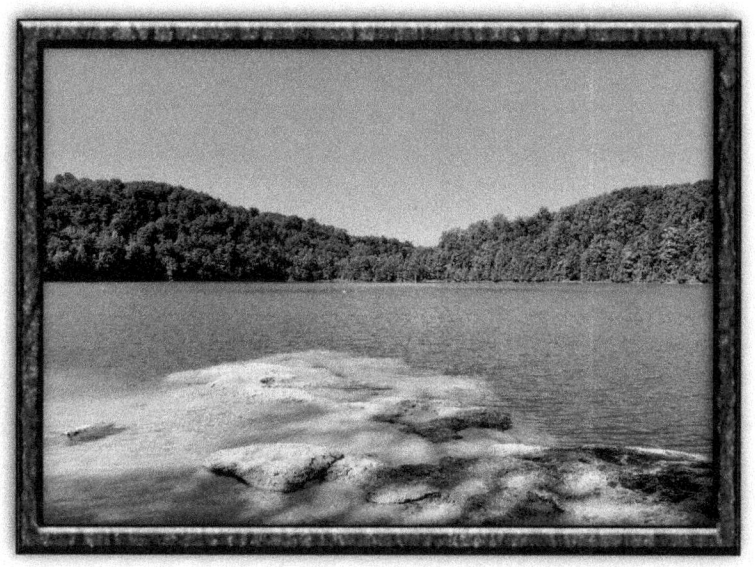

Green Lakes State Park

Location

Green Lakes State Park is located just outside of Syracuse, in Onondaga County, making it part of Central New York, but often considered within the broader region of Western New York due to its proximity to the Finger Lakes area.

The park is situated in the village of Fayetteville, approximately 10 miles east of downtown Syracuse. This strategic location makes it easily accessible for those coming from Syracuse, as well as from other parts of Western New York or even travelers from further afield looking to explore the natural beauty of the region. Green Lakes State Park is nestled near the eastern edge of the Finger Lakes, adding to its allure with its unique glacial lakes, surrounded by lush, old-growth forest.

Ryans Notes:

    This park has a lot of parking and many hills to walk through. As we go into the park itself we had to walk up the hill to get to where they have an RV park, we went through the park to a walkway that goes around the whole lake, in was a nice walkway because it was shaded enough to keep you cool, but also your able to see everything around you. As we walked we found the beach that everyone was on, but we just kept walking. On this side there was a narrow walkway with a large rock in the water that people were going out to and taking pictures. Ryan asked me to take a picture of him, so I did, though I was concerned with his balance but he had no problems with it. Ryan saw a steep hill and wanted to go up it so I could take a picture up the hill then went back down the hill on his but. He brushed himself off and kept on walking. We ended up walking around both lakes up and down the hills and back to the car, heading back home to Amherst.

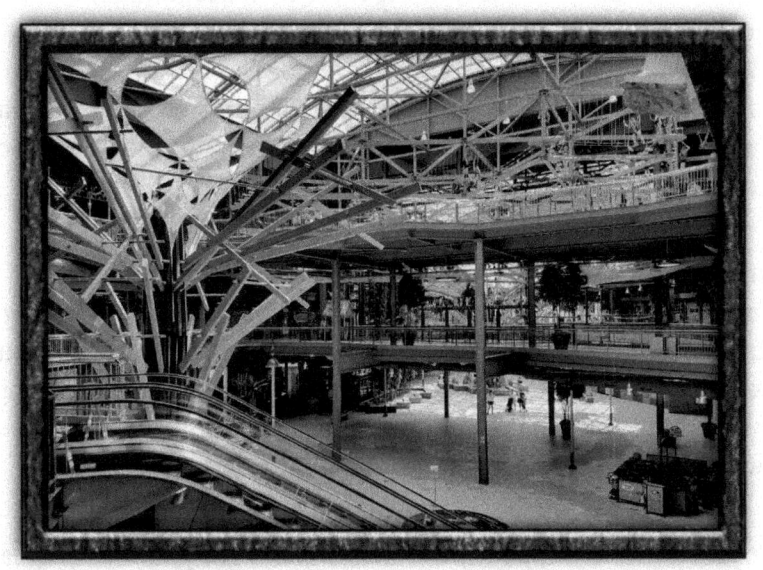

Destiny USA Mall

Location

Destiny USA Mall is situated in the city of Syracuse, in Onondaga County, New York. Although Syracuse is often considered part of Central New York, its inclusion in broader discussions about Western New York is due to its proximity to the Finger Lakes region and its cultural and economic ties to the area.

The mall is located on the shore of Onondaga Lake, making it a prominent feature in the Syracuse skyline. It's easily accessible from Interstate 81 and close to the New York State Thruway (I-90), positioning it as a central hub for shopping, dining, and entertainment for residents of Syracuse and visitors from across Western New York and beyond.

History

The story of Destiny USA Mall is one of transformation, ambition, and the economic evolution of Syracuse. The site where the mall now stands was once nothing more than a landfill known as Marley Scrap Yard, surrounded by oil tanks in an area ironically nicknamed "Oil City." The Pyramid Companies saw the potential in this blighted industrial landscape, envisioning a retail giant that would not only change the physical skyline but also the economic landscape of Syracuse.

Initially opened in 1990 as Carousel Center, the mall was named for the historic carousel that became one of its signature features. From its inception, Carousel Center was ambitious, aiming to be a multi-level shopping experience with a mix of upscale and discount retailers. However, it wasn't without its detractors, facing competition from other local malls and criticism over its impact on downtown Syracuse's revival.

The transformation into Destiny USA began in 2007 when plans for a massive expansion were unveiled. The goal was to create one of the largest malls in the United States, incorporating green technology, entertainment, and a diverse retail offering. This expansion was fraught with legal battles, debates over environmental concerns, tax incentives, and the use of RFID technology for monitoring consumer habits. Despite these obstacles, Destiny USA officially opened its expanded form in 2012, redefining what a shopping mall could be by including attractions like an IMAX theater and a variety of dining and entertainment options.

Destiny USA has had a profound economic impact on Syracuse, drawing millions of visitors and creating jobs. However, it has also sparked discussions about its effect on local commerce, the sustainability of mega-malls, and how it reshapes urban consumer culture. Over the years, challenges have been plentiful, from the general decline in traditional retail to specific issues like crime and security within the mall itself. Destiny USA has had to adapt, continuously evolving its tenant mix, introducing new entertainment options, and shifting its identity from solely a shopping destination to a broader entertainment and lifestyle center.

In recent times, Destiny USA reflects the broader challenges facing American malls, with store closures and the need to innovate in response to changing consumer behaviors. Yet, its history is a testament to the vision of reclaiming and repurposing urban land for public use, illustrating the complexities and possibilities of urban redevelopment in the modern era.

Terrain

Visitors to Destiny USA Mall will encounter a terrain that's predominantly urban and indoor, tailored for shopping, dining, and entertainment:

Indoor Environment: The primary terrain at Destiny USA is the vast, multi-level interior of the mall itself. The floors are mostly flat, covered with polished tile or carpet, accommodating easy navigation for shoppers, strollers, and those with mobility aids. The mall's design includes escalators, elevators, and wide corridors to facilitate movement between its various levels and destinations.

Outdoor Areas: While much of the experience is indoors, there are outdoor spaces associated with the mall. The entrance areas might feature paved walkways or plazas where one can find seasonal decorations or outdoor seating. These areas provide a transition from the urban street to the mall's interior.

Waterfront Access: Destiny USA is uniquely positioned along Onondaga Lake. Although the mall itself doesn't extend directly to the water, there's a connection to the lake through nearby trails and a small park area. Visitors can experience a change in terrain here, from the mall's hard surfaces to the softer, sometimes grassy or pebbled areas near the water, offering a place for relaxation or outdoor activities.

Parking and Access: The mall's parking facilities are extensive, with both surface lots and multi-story parking structures. The terrain here includes ramps, stairs, and elevators for accessing different levels of parking. The ground can be asphalt or concrete, with painted lines for parking spaces and pedestrian walkways.

Seasonal Considerations: The indoor environment of Destiny USA remains consistent regardless of weather, but for those accessing the mall from outside, seasonal changes can affect the experience. Winter might bring snow or ice in parking areas, requiring caution, while summer could mean enjoying outdoor events or simply the lake view under warmer skies.

Entertainment Zones: Within the mall, there are areas specifically designed for entertainment, like the Canyon, which simulates an outdoor environment with rock formations and waterfalls, providing a different feel from the standard mall terrain.

Accessibility: Destiny USA is designed with accessibility in mind, ensuring that the terrain, both inside and around the mall, is navigable for people with disabilities. This includes ramps, accessible restrooms, and clear pathways.

Overall, while Destiny USA's terrain is largely that of an urban shopping complex, its integration with outdoor spaces and its unique indoor features ensure a varied experience for visitors, blending the convenience of mall shopping with the natural beauty of its lakeside location.

Ryan's Notes:

This was our final weekend trip of the year. We first started our day at Density U.S. Once we got into the parking lot we noticed this place was huge. In some parts of the mall it was 5 stories tall are connected to a hotel. We had lunch at Johnny Rockets, which is a 50s restaurant. In the mall there is a small zoo, an amusement park, R.C. car racing as well as a Nascar go cart place. I got excited to drive a car. The people at the go cart place were extremely helpful and friendly, I highly recommend checking it out when you stop there. I went through the mall with Jamie and since we still had time left we went to the Onondaga lake park. Jamie decided to sit by the lake to watch the sun set. So I went walking round the lake, Jamie called me when I was walking seeing if I needed her I told her there was a the lake on the one side and on the other side next to me was the highway, so I kept walking until I stopped at a gas station and asked the lady to please put the address in a text message to Jamie so she could get me. She did, then I started talking with her about my disability and what I do. Jamie came and went into the gas station. Jamie thanked the lady and she asked about Ryan and was amazed what Ryan was able to do. She went on to explain she had a son with a disability and was concerned what would happen to him when she was gone. Jamie explains that Ryan was able to do the things he could do because of the People Inc. programs. For Jamie it was amazing to see first hand how Ryan touches people's lives. Jamie came back into the car asking what I said and did. My eyes widened. I thought I did something wrong and then she told me what happend. And if I did something wrong why didnt she call the cops?

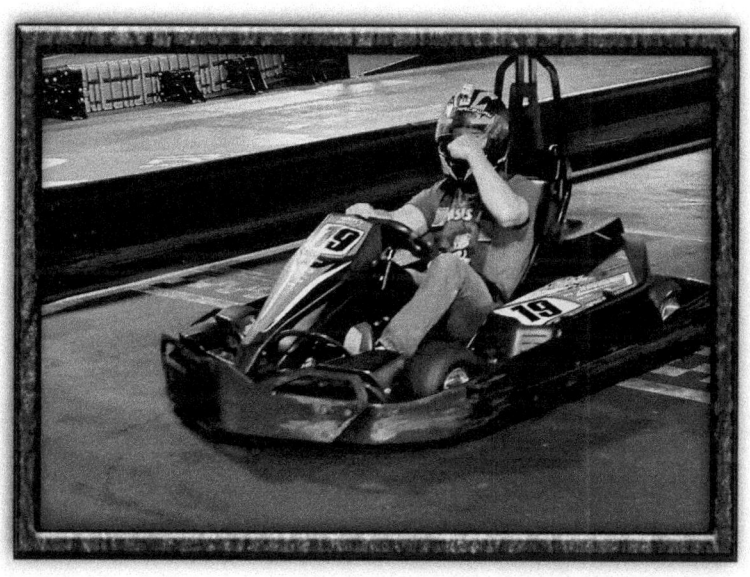

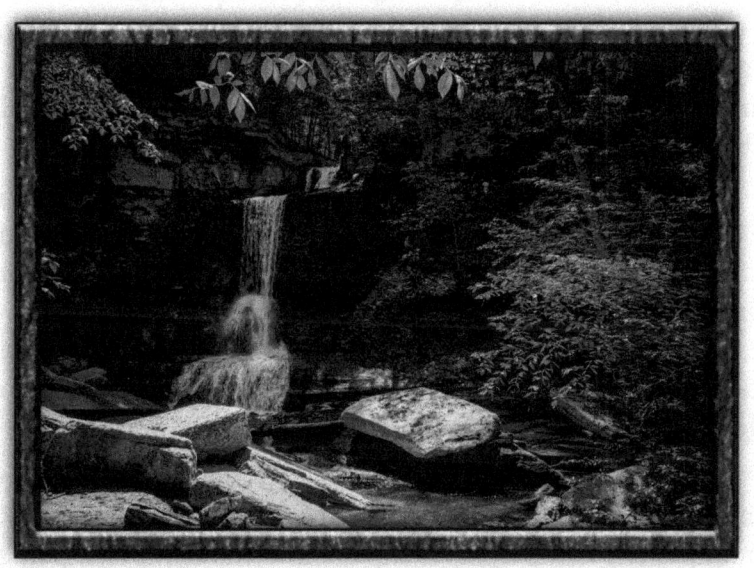

Fillmore Glen State Park

Location

Fillmore Glen State Park is located in the Finger Lakes region of Western New York, specifically in Cayuga County.

The park is nestled just outside the village of Moravia, roughly 30 miles south of Auburn and about 20 miles north of Ithaca. This positioning places it in a scenic part of Western New York, known for its natural beauty, with the park offering access to the unique gorge, waterfalls, and forested landscapes characteristic of the Finger Lakes area. Its location makes it both a serene retreat from urban life and a convenient destination for outdoor enthusiasts looking to explore the region's natural wonders.

History

The history of Fillmore Glen State Park is rich with natural evolution and human influence, telling a story of conservation, community, and connection to one of America's former presidents:

Originally, the area where Fillmore Glen now stands was known for its abundant plant life and was used by local Native American communities, though specific historical records of their use are sparse. The natural beauty of the area, with its gorge and waterfalls, had long been recognized by those who lived nearby.

The park's development into what we recognize today began in the early 20th century. In 1925, New York State acquired the land, initially naming it "Glen State Park." It was later renamed Fillmore Glen State Park in honor of Millard Fillmore, the 13th President of the United States, who was born nearby in Locke, New York. The park includes a replica of his childhood cabin, tying its history to Fillmore's legacy.

The park saw significant development during the Great Depression through the efforts of the Civilian Conservation Corps (CCC). From 1934 to 1938, CCC workers constructed many of the park's enduring features, including stone walls, bridges, and trails, which have become part of the park's charm and historical value. Their work not only beautified the park but also made it more accessible to the public, enhancing its recreational potential.

Over the decades, Fillmore Glen has evolved from a raw natural area into a cherished state park, serving as a sanctuary for outdoor activities like hiking, camping, and nature observation. The park has hosted various events, drawing visitors to experience its natural wonders, from the five waterfalls along Dry Creek (originally Dry Brook) to the dense, cool woods of the gorge.

The history of Fillmore Glen State Park reflects a broader narrative of how natural landscapes can be preserved and celebrated through state initiatives, community involvement, and historical appreciation, ensuring that its beauty can be enjoyed by generations to come.

Terrain

Visitors to Fillmore Glen State Park will find themselves immersed in a landscape that combines the rugged beauty of a gorge with more serene woodland areas:

Gorge and Waterfalls: The park's most distinctive feature is the gorge carved by Dry Creek, featuring five waterfalls. The terrain here involves trails that wind along the creek, sometimes climbing up or down the gorge's sides. These paths can be steep, with rocky steps, wooden or stone staircases, and narrow passages that require careful footing, especially when wet or icy.

Hiking Trails: There are several trails, varying from easy to moderate in difficulty. The Gorge Trail, for instance, offers an intimate experience with the natural rock formations, waterfalls, and the creek itself, often involving elevation changes. Other trails like the North Rim Trail provide a less strenuous but still engaging hike through forested areas with occasional views down into the gorge.

Forest and Woodland: Outside the immediate gorge, the terrain shifts to a typical woodland setting with flat to gently rolling paths. Here, the ground is covered with leaves, pine needles, or sometimes gravel, offering a more relaxed walking experience through mature forests. These areas are ideal for bird watching, wildlife spotting, or simply enjoying the peace of nature.

Campsites and Picnic Areas: The camping and picnic areas are set on relatively flat, grassy, or graveled spots, making them accessible and comfortable for setting up tents or enjoying meals. These spaces are designed to blend with the natural environment while providing ease of use.

Seasonal Variations: The park's terrain transforms with the seasons. In spring, the ground can be damp, and the waterfalls are at their fullest. Summer brings lush greenery and potentially higher water levels in the creek. Autumn paints the park in vibrant colors, with leaves covering paths, and winter might see some trails under snow or ice, altering the hiking experience, with certain areas possibly closed for safety.

Historical Structures: The CCC's influence is visible in the stone work, making parts of the trail not only a physical journey but also a walk through history, where the terrain includes man-made elements that have become part of the natural landscape.

Accessibility: While much of the park offers a rugged outdoor experience, there are efforts to make parts of Fillmore Glen accessible to those with mobility challenges, although the natural state of the park means some areas remain less accessible.

Visitors should come prepared for a diverse terrain that challenges and rewards with its natural beauty, requiring appropriate footwear and an adventurous spirit to fully enjoy the park's offerings.

Ryan's Notes:

When Jamie and I first arrived, there was a cabin so we walked in. Jamie of course and took my picture. We left the building and walked into the field where there was a playground, past that was the hills to walk on. We noticed that there were construction workers trying to fix the erosion from the past year. As we started to walk we saw the river beneath us and kept on the paths which in some areas got narrow and some paths were wide, Ryan as usual went ahead and was able to walk through the entire park, went back to the playground, started talking with a family he just met, while Jamie was still making her way down. Ryan looked up to me and said what took you so long. We went over the bridge and headed back to the car and onward to Syracuse to our next adventure.

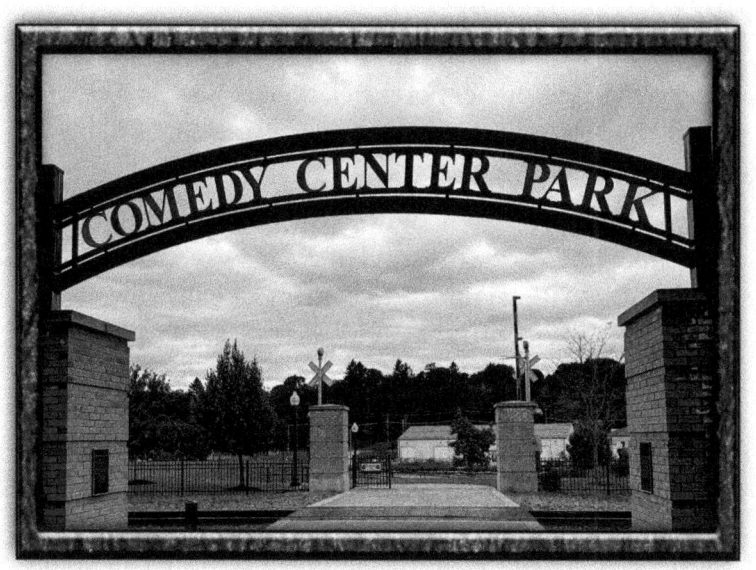

Jamestown Comedy Central Park

Location

Jamestown Comedy Central Park is located in the city of Jamestown, within Chautauqua County in the southwestern part of New York State.

This park is right in the heart of Jamestown's downtown area, making it easily accessible for both locals and visitors. Jamestown is approximately 70 miles southwest of Buffalo and about 40 miles southeast of Erie, Pennsylvania. This location situates the park near Lake Chautauqua and not far from the Pennsylvania border, offering a unique blend of urban and natural environments. It's strategically placed next to the National Comedy Center, enhancing its significance as a cultural hub in Western New York dedicated to celebrating comedy.

Ryan G. Young

History

The history of Jamestown Comedy Central Park is closely intertwined with the development of the National Comedy Center and the city's homage to one of its most famous residents, Lucille Ball. Here's how it unfolded:

Jamestown has long been known as the birthplace of Lucille Ball, a legendary figure in the world of comedy and television. The idea of creating a park dedicated to comedy in Jamestown was part of a broader vision to honor Ball's legacy and turn the city into a destination for comedy enthusiasts.

The park's creation was catalyzed by the establishment of the National Comedy Center in 2018, which itself was a transformation of the earlier Lucille Ball-Desi Arnaz Museum. The National Comedy Center, conceived with the aim of preserving and celebrating the history of comedy in America, naturally extended its influence to the surrounding area, leading to the development of Comedy Central Park.

This park, often referred to simply as "Comedy Park," was designed as an outdoor space where visitors could continue their comedic journey started within the museum walls. It serves as a public space for events, performances, and community gatherings, enhancing the cultural offerings of Jamestown. The park's design and programming reflect themes of comedy, with art installations, performance stages, and spaces for outdoor activities that align with the Center's mission.

The park has also been a venue for various events during the annual Lucille Ball Comedy Festival, drawing comedians and comedy fans alike to celebrate humor in a setting that blends the natural beauty of Jamestown with its comedic heritage. Over time, it has become not just a physical space but a symbol of Jamestown's commitment to its cultural identity, encapsulated by Ball's influence and the broader narrative of American comedy.

The history of Jamestown Comedy Central Park, therefore, is a story of community pride, cultural preservation, and the transformation of a city's identity through its most celebrated daughter, making it a unique addition to Western New York's cultural landscape.

Terrain

Visitors to Jamestown Comedy Central Park can expect a terrain that blends urban convenience with a touch of whimsy, reflective of its comedic theme:

Urban Park Setting: The park is situated in the heart of downtown Jamestown, meaning the terrain is primarily that of an urban park. The ground is mostly level, with paved or concrete pathways that make for easy walking. These paths are designed to accommodate strollers, wheelchairs, and those with mobility aids, ensuring accessibility.

Open Spaces: There are open grassy areas where events, performances, or casual picnicking might occur. These spaces offer a soft, green contrast to the surrounding cityscape, providing a place for relaxation or community activities.

Art Installations and Features: The park includes various art installations themed around comedy, which might involve interactive or visual elements that could alter the usual park terrain. For instance, there might be sculptures, benches with comedic quotes, or temporary setups for festivals, slightly changing the landscape.

Performance Areas: A stage or platform for performances is likely part of the terrain, possibly with an amphitheater-like setup for seating. This area might have a different surface, like wood or raised concrete, to accommodate shows and events.

Seasonal Adaptations: In winter, the park might see snow, necessitating shoveled paths or areas cleared for events. Summer might bring temporary installations or structures for festivals. The terrain thus adapts to seasonal programming, with potential changes in layout or additional features like tents or barriers for events.

Landscaping: The park's landscaping includes trees, shrubs, and perhaps flower beds, offering shaded spots and adding to the park's aesthetic appeal. These natural elements might frame paths or create cozy nooks for visitors.

Connection to the National Comedy Center: The park seamlessly integrates with the National Comedy Center, meaning the transition from indoors to outdoors is smooth, with pathways or entry points designed for ease of access.

Overall, the terrain at Jamestown Comedy Central Park is user-friendly, designed to enhance the visitor's experience of both the city's urban environment and its celebration of comedy, making it a place where laughter and leisure are equally accessible.

Ryan's Notes:

This was one of our last trips, unfortunately the comedy museum was closed but we decided to check out the park behind the museum. It started off by the railway station. You go through the archway into the park. When you walk through there are signs explaining different interesting facts about the area. As you walk you go under the bridge to an aqueduct. There is another walkway that goes into the town. We ended up doing both walkways. This day was sunny, cloudy and raining on and off. We ended walking to this little food shop mom/pop shop for lunch. The food was amazing. It was starting to get nasty so we ended up walking through the town back to the car and headed home.

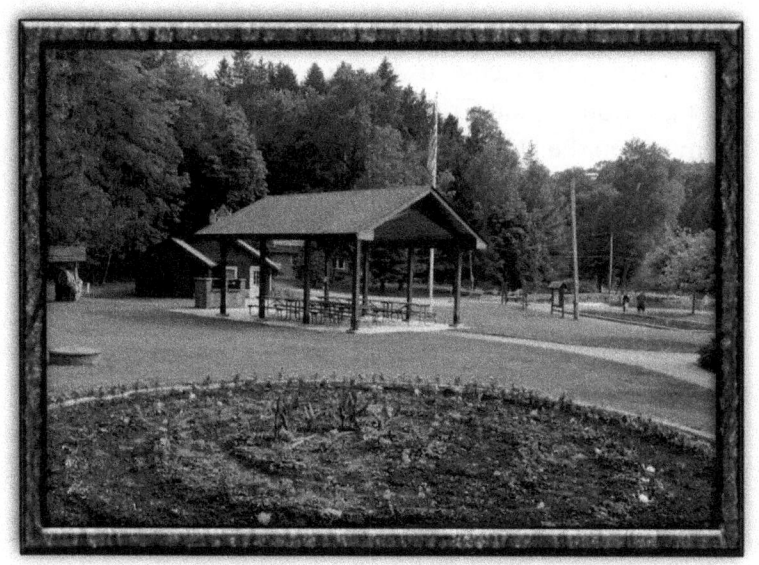

Powder Mills Park

Location

Powder Mills Park is located in the town of Pittsford, within Monroe County, in the western part of New York State.

The park is situated southeast of Rochester, accessible from Route 96 South of Bushnell's Basin near Interstate 490. Its strategic location makes it a convenient recreational spot for residents of Rochester and surrounding areas, providing an escape into nature without straying far from urban conveniences. Pittsford is known for its charming village center, and Powder Mills Park adds to the area's appeal with its natural beauty and recreational offerings.

History

The history of Powder Mills Park intertwines with both the natural landscape and the industrial legacy of Western New York. Initially, the land was home to the Seneca Nation of the Iroquois Confederacy, who made use of the area's natural resources. However, the story that gives the park its name begins in the early 20th century with the establishment of the DuPont Company's powder mill. Recognizing the secluded site's potential and its access to the power of the Irondequoit Creek, E.I. du Pont de Nemours and Company set up the DuPont Powder Mills in 1905. This facility became a key player in the production of black powder, serving the needs of construction, mining, and military operations during a time when such materials were in high demand.

After World War II, with the decline in the use of black powder, the operations at the DuPont plant came to a close in the late 1940s. This marked the beginning of a new chapter for the land. In 1961, Monroe County saw the opportunity to transform this site from an industrial area back into a natural retreat for public enjoyment. The land was acquired, and Powder Mills Park was born, reflecting a broader movement in the post-war era to create public spaces from former industrial sites.

The park's development over the subsequent years focused on preserving its natural beauty while acknowledging its historical significance. Trails were laid out, often following the old mill races, providing visitors with a tangible link to the past. Picnic areas, fishing spots, and wildlife observation points were established, making the park a haven for outdoor enthusiasts. Remnants of the powder mill, now integrated into the landscape, serve as silent educators about the area's industrial history alongside its ecological richness.

Today, Powder Mills Park stands as a testament to the shift from industry to conservation, a place where the past and present coexist. It's not only a recreational spot but also an educational site where one can learn about the industrial heritage of the region alongside its natural history, making it a unique destination in Western New York.

Terrain

Visitors to Powder Mills Park will encounter a varied and engaging terrain that balances natural beauty with historical remnants:

Wooded Trails: Much of the park is covered by mature forests, with trails that wind through these woods. The ground here can be soft with leaves, pine needles, or occasionally roots and rocks, offering an authentic hiking experience. These trails vary from wide, easy paths to narrow, more adventurous routes, catering to different levels of exploration.

Creek Side Paths: Irondequoit Creek runs through the park, providing a scenic backdrop with its banks offering both flat and slightly rugged terrain. The paths near the creek can be gravel, dirt, or grass, with some areas featuring small stone steps or bridges to cross the water or navigate changes in elevation. The creek's presence makes for a serene environment, ideal for fishing or simply enjoying the sounds of flowing water.

Historical Features: The remnants of the old DuPont Powder Mills subtly influence the terrain. Visitors might come across leveled areas where buildings once stood, now integrated into the park's landscape, or see stone foundations that have become part of the natural scenery. These historical elements add a unique texture to the park's topography.

Open Areas: There are clearings and picnic spots with flat, grassy areas where visitors can enjoy open spaces. These areas are well-maintained, providing a contrast to the wooded sections and offering spaces for games, relaxation, or community events.

Elevation Changes: While the park doesn't feature dramatic elevation changes, there are gentle slopes and inclines that add a bit of challenge to the hiking experience, particularly around the creek where the land naturally undulates.

Seasonal Variations: The terrain changes with the seasons; autumn brings a carpet of leaves that can make paths slippery, winter might see snow covering the trails, altering the walking experience, and spring and summer offer blooming flora and lush greenery.

Accessibility: Efforts have been made to ensure some areas are accessible, with wider paths and smoother surfaces for those with mobility challenges, although the natural state of much of the park means some areas might be less accessible.

Ryan G. Young

The terrain at Powder Mills Park invites visitors into a world where history and nature converge, offering both the tranquility of wooded walks and the intrigue of exploring a site with a rich industrial past now reclaimed by nature.

Ryan's Notes:

This park is close to Eastview mall. This park is actually a fish hatchery. The weather was still icky out but we still wanted to walk. So we walked around the fish ponds looking at the fish. There were different sizes and different ages. Once we looked at the fish we kept walking up the hill continuing to go through the park and ventured into a path that lead into the woods. We walked and walked until the clouds got very dark and Jamie said it was time to go, so we turned around and headed back to the car and it started to rain. By the time we got back to the car we were soaked. Still it was a very interesting place to visit.

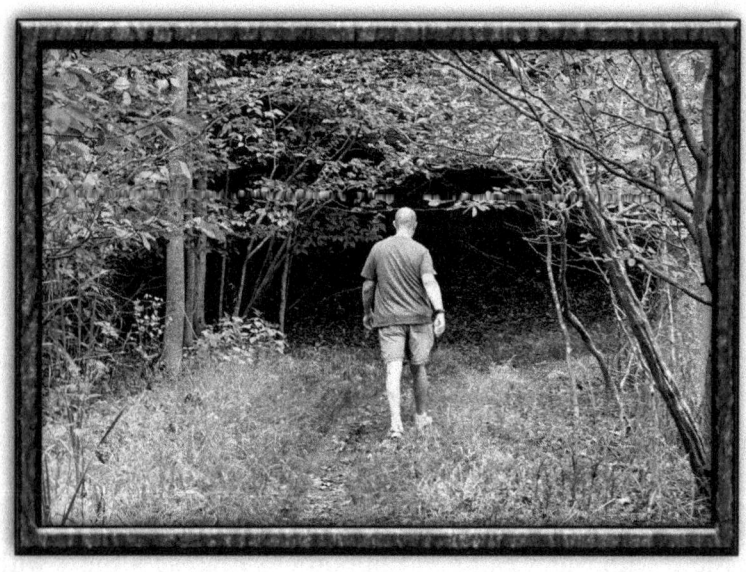

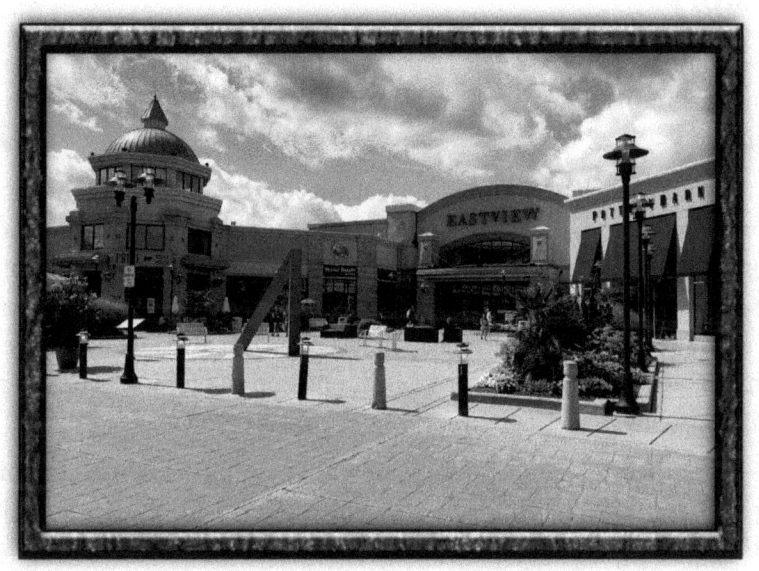

Eastview Mall

Location

Eastview Mall is located in the town of Victor, within Ontario County, in Western New York.

This major shopping destination is situated just off New York State Thruway (Interstate 90) Exit 45, making it highly accessible for those coming from Rochester, which is about 20 miles northwest, or from other parts of the region including the Finger Lakes area. Victor is known for its proximity to the Finger Lakes wine region and for being part of the Greater Rochester area, blending suburban charm with access to urban amenities. Eastview Mall serves as a shopping hub for residents and visitors alike, drawing from a wide geographical area due to its strategic location and extensive retail offerings.

History

The history of Eastview Mall reflects the transformation of rural farmland into one of Western New York's premier shopping destinations:

Eastview Mall was built on what was once 73 acres of Ontario County farmland, marking a significant shift in the landscape and economy of Victor. Its construction began in the late 1960s, with the mall officially opening its doors in 1971. This development was spearheaded by Wilmorite Properties, a local real estate and development company known for its influence on the region's commercial landscape.

From the outset, Eastview Mall was an ambitious project, aiming to serve not just Victor but the entire Metro-Rochester area. Its initial tenants included Sibley's and Sears, which were major department stores at the time. Just a year later, in 1972, it expanded to include McCurdy's, further establishing its reputation as a shopping destination.

Over the years, Eastview Mall has undergone several expansions, each reflecting changes in retail trends and consumer habits:

A significant expansion added a new wing with additional stores, including JCPenney and Lord & Taylor, doubling the mall's size to over 1.3 million square feet.

2003 Enhancements: Another expansion focused on lifestyle and dining, introducing upscale stores and restaurants near the main entrance, enhancing the mall's appeal as a place for both shopping and leisure.

The mall has seen the evolution of its anchor stores with Sibley's becoming Kaufmann's and then Macy's, McCurdy's turning into The Bon-Ton and then Von Maur, and the departure of Lord & Taylor in 2020 due to the economic impact of the COVID-19 pandemic. Each of these changes has been a part of adapting to the retail environment.

Community Impact: Eastview Mall has had a profound impact on Victor, turning it from a sleepy farming community into a retail mecca. It has contributed to local employment, tax revenues, and has become a cultural and social hub for the area, often hosting community events and seasonal celebrations.

The history of Eastview Mall is not just about commerce but also about how a mall can become a central part of a community's identity, adapting over time to meet the needs and desires of its visitors while leaving a lasting mark on the development of Victor and the broader Rochester area.

Terrain

Visitors to Eastview Mall will experience a terrain that is quintessentially urban and designed for ease of shopping and navigation:

The primary terrain within Eastview Mall is flat and smooth, with polished tile or carpeted floors throughout the shopping areas. This indoor environment is climate-controlled, ensuring a comfortable walk regardless of the weather outside. The mall's design includes wide corridors, escalators, elevators, and stairs to facilitate movement between its various levels and shops.

The exterior of the mall features paved parking lots and sidewalks. These areas are level, with painted lines to guide parking and pedestrian traffic. During certain times of the year, such as holiday seasons, there might be additional outdoor setups for events or temporary attractions, which can slightly alter the usual terrain with added structures or decorations.

Around the mall, there is some landscaping with grass, shrubs, and trees, providing aesthetic appeal and sometimes seating areas for outdoor breaks. These green spaces are maintained but are minimal compared to the vast indoor shopping area.

Eastview Mall prides itself on being accessible, with ramps, automatic doors, and clear signage to aid those with mobility issues or disabilities. The flat terrain inside ensures that moving from store to store is straightforward for everyone.

While the indoor environment remains consistent, outdoor areas can be affected by weather. Snow removal in winter keeps the parking lots and walkways clear, but visitors might need to navigate a bit of snow or slush. In contrast, summer might mean more outdoor activities or events, potentially altering the usual outdoor setup.

The mall includes multi-level parking structures where the terrain involves ramps and levels for parking. These areas require a bit more navigation, but they are designed with ease of access in mind, including elevators for those who need them.

The terrain at Eastview Mall is designed with the shopper in mind, focusing on comfort, accessibility, and convenience, making it an ideal environment for a day of retail therapy or leisure in Western New York.

Ryan"s Notes:

This was our first time in Rochester, the weather was cloudy with the potential to rain so we decided to go and explore the mall. The place was huge and took awhile to walk through we had lunch there and had a good time , we then decided since the weather was ok we would go to powermill park.

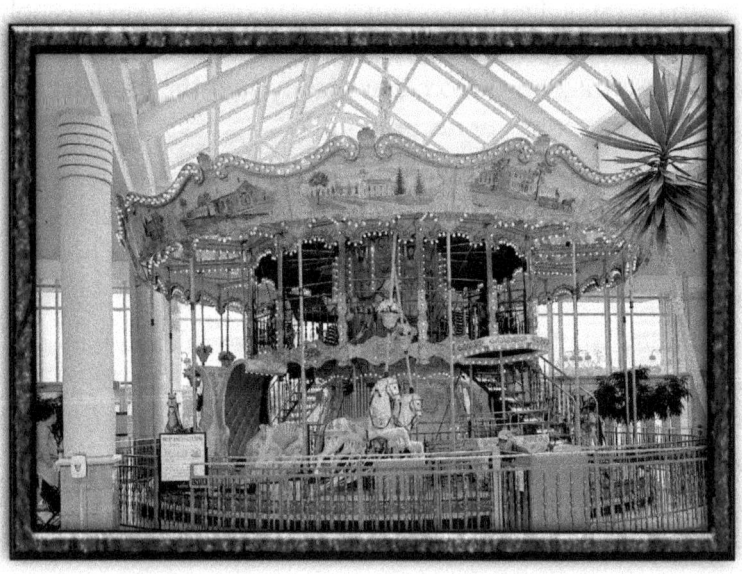

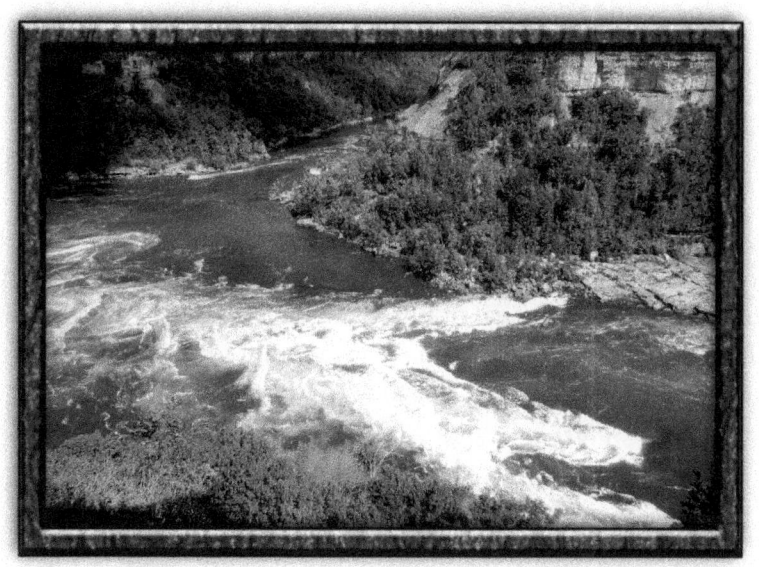

Whirlpool State Park

Location

Whirlpool State Park is found in Niagara County, Western New York, near the city of Niagara Falls.

This park is directly adjacent to the Niagara Gorge and the Niagara River, providing stunning views of the Niagara Whirlpool. It's situated just south of the famous Niagara Falls, making it part of the greater Niagara Falls State Park area. The proximity to Niagara Falls means it's easily accessible for tourists visiting the falls, and it's approximately 20 miles northwest of Buffalo, placing it in one of the most scenic and visited regions of Western New York.

History

The history of Whirlpool State Park is as dynamic as the waters that flow through it, intertwining with the geological marvels and cultural evolution of the Niagara River and Falls. The Niagara Whirlpool itself, the park's namesake, was sculpted over millennia by the relentless carving of the Niagara River through the bedrock of the Niagara Escarpment. This natural phenomenon, where the river dramatically bends and swirls, has been a landmark of awe for countless generations.

Long before European settlers set foot in the area, the Seneca and Neutral Nations, among others, held the whirlpool in high regard. It was a place of fishing, a marker in their territory, and possibly held spiritual significance, embodying the power and beauty of nature. With the arrival of Europeans, the Niagara Falls region, including the whirlpool, became a focal point for exploration and tourism, drawing visitors eager to witness one of nature's most spectacular displays.

The official establishment of Whirlpool State Park in 1928 was part of a broader initiative to preserve and promote the natural wonders of the Niagara region. As tourism boomed, there was a growing recognition of the need to protect these landscapes while allowing public access. The park's creation was a step towards ensuring that the natural beauty of the Niagara Gorge and its whirlpool could be enjoyed by future generations.

In the early 20th century, an aerial ropeway was built over the whirlpool, providing visitors with an unparalleled view of this natural wonder, though it no longer operates today. Over the years, the park has been the setting for various historical attractions and daredevil attempts, adding a rich tapestry of human endeavor to its natural history.

Today, Whirlpool State Park is both a conservation area and a recreational space, with trails, staircases, and overlooks designed to offer safe exploration of its rugged terrain. It stands as a testament to the balance between enjoyment and preservation, a place where one can witness the raw power of nature alongside the human efforts to respect and protect it.

Terrain

Visitors to Whirlpool State Park will encounter a terrain that reflects the dramatic natural beauty of the Niagara Gorge:

Gorge and Cliffs: The park's most defining feature is the steep walls of the Niagara Gorge, offering breathtaking views of the whirlpool below. The terrain here includes cliff edges with safety railings, providing secure vantage points but also requiring caution. Trails along these edges can involve steep ascents or descents, with many steps carved into the rock or built from wood or stone.

Hiking Trails: There are several trails within the park, ranging from easy walks to more challenging hikes. The Devil's Hole Trail, for example, winds through the woods and along the gorge, offering both flat sections and steep, uneven parts with natural obstacles like rocks and roots. This diversity in trail difficulty caters to various levels of hiking enthusiasts.

Staircases and Lookouts: To navigate the vertical changes, the park features numerous staircases, some quite long, that lead down into the gorge or up to observation points. These structures are integral for experiencing the full scope of the park's beauty but require a good level of fitness to traverse.

River Access: The park does not provide direct access to the Niagara River at the whirlpool due to the sheer cliffs, but there are spots where one can get closer to the water's edge, particularly at lower levels of the gorge. Here, the terrain can be rocky, potentially slippery, and requires careful navigation.

Seasonal Changes: The terrain's experience changes with the seasons. Winter can bring ice and snow, making some trails treacherous or closed, while spring and fall might see water making paths slippery or enhancing the park's natural beauty with vibrant foliage. Summer offers the best conditions for exploration but can be hot at the top of the gorge.

Natural Surfaces: Much of the park's ground is natural - dirt, gravel, rock - contrasting with the urban environment of nearby Niagara Falls. This means that footwear with good traction is advisable for tackling the varied and sometimes rugged terrain.

Accessibility: While the park strives to be accessible, the rugged nature of the terrain means that some areas are less suited for those with mobility issues, although there are efforts to provide accessible overlooks for panoramic views without the need for extensive hiking.

Whirlpool State Park offers an adventure where the terrain challenges visitors to engage with the landscape, rewarding them with some of the most spectacular views in Western New York.

Ryan's Notes:

It was a bright sunny day. We got out of the car near the electrical power station. As we walked into the park each side of the path trees were covered, keeping it shaded. Next to the paths are cliffs heading into the gorge. Also known as devils hole. As we walked down the paths we passed the conservation station. Jamie talked to the educators and they told her to go down the gorge paths 350 steps down. I decided to go down the steps, Jamie decided to wait up top. As Jamie was waiting she couldn't see me so decided to go down the stairs on a sore ankle. So I met her on the bottom and she was nervous to go back up so I kept encouraging to go and she was so excited that she made it back up.

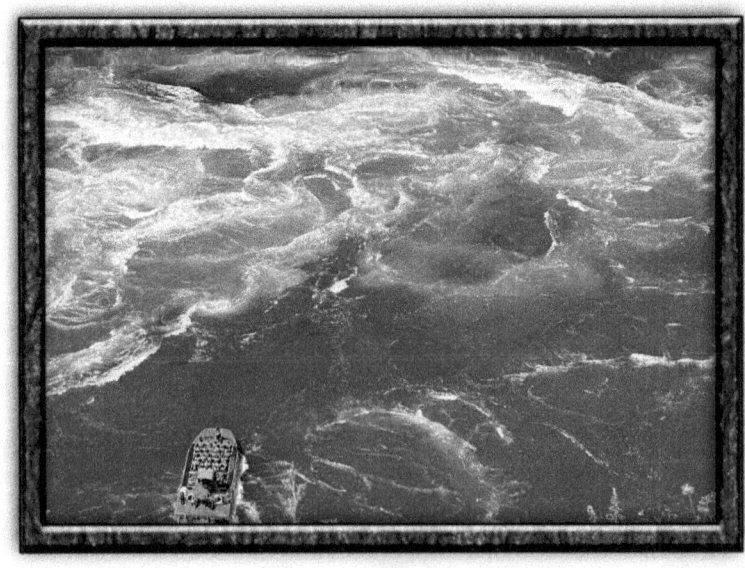

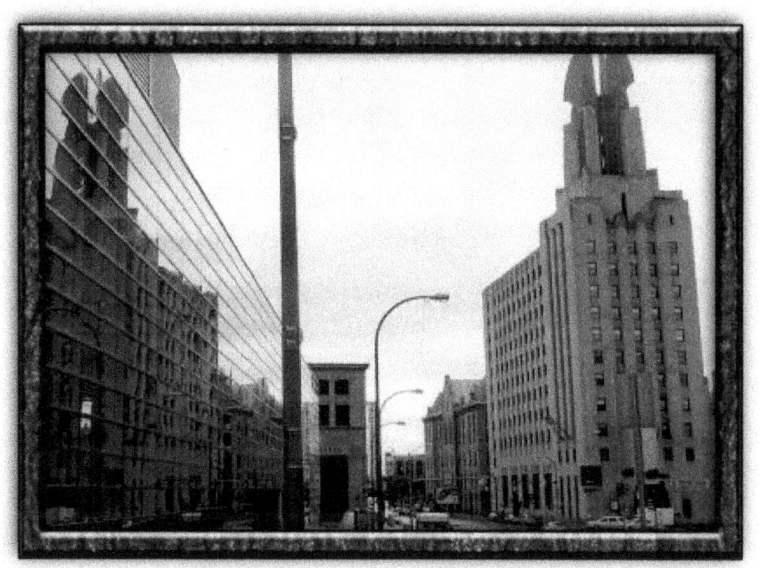

Rochester Square

Location

Rochester Square is situated in the heart of Rochester, within Monroe County, in Western New York.

Rochester, known for its contributions to photography, optics, and education, is the third-largest city in New York State. Rochester Square, if it's conceptualized as a central or notable area within the city, would be near other landmarks like the Eastman Theatre, the Genesee River, and close to the cultural and business districts of downtown. This location makes it easily accessible from major routes like Interstate 490, placing it in a vibrant part of Western New York, surrounded by historical architecture and modern urban amenities.

History

The history of Rochester Square, envisioned as a central or historically significant area in Rochester, is profoundly linked to the city's own development. Rochester's narrative begins in the late 18th century, with significant growth following the completion of the Erie Canal in 1825, which catapulted the city into a commercial powerhouse, known as the "Flour City" for its milling prowess. What might now be referred to as Rochester Square would have emerged as the heart of this burgeoning city, centered around the Genesee River and the bustling activity of trade.

As Rochester grew, the area around Main Street and East Avenue became synonymous with the city's commercial, cultural, and civic life. This part of downtown saw the rise of impressive architecture from the Greek Revival to Art Deco, with landmarks like the Times Square Building standing as testaments to the city's architectural evolution. These buildings were not just commercial spaces but also hubs for cultural activities, housing theaters, banks, and later, significant cultural institutions like the Eastman School of Music

Rochester Square would have been a witness to pivotal moments in American social history. It was here that figures like Frederick Douglass spoke, contributing to Rochester's reputation as a center for abolitionist thought. The area also played a role in the women's suffrage movement, with figures like Susan B. Anthony advocating for change within its bounds.

The modern era brought its own transformations. Like many urban centers, Rochester Square might have seen its identity shift with urban renewal, the rise of suburban shopping, and economic fluctuations. Yet, in recent decades, there's been a concerted effort towards revitalization, aiming to make downtown Rochester not just a place of commerce but a vibrant community hub. This includes preserving historical buildings, introducing new residential and entertainment options, and fostering local business growth to rekindle the area's allure.

The history of Rochester Square, then, is a microcosm of Rochester's journey from a canal-side settlement to a city with deep roots in American industry, culture, and social reform, reflecting both its challenges and its enduring spirit of renewal.

Terrain

Visitors to Rochester Square, assuming it's a central or significant part of downtown Rochester, will encounter a terrain that reflects the city's urban landscape:

Urban Streets: The primary terrain in this area would be city streets, lined with sidewalks made of concrete or brick. These sidewalks are generally flat, accommodating pedestrian traffic, but might include occasional inclines or steps where the city's topography varies or where buildings step up or down to meet the street level.

Public Spaces and Plazas: Rochester Square likely includes public squares or plazas where the terrain is more open, often paved with materials like stone or concrete, designed for events, markets, or simply for people to gather. These areas might feature benches, planters, or public art, offering a break from the urban grid.

Historical and Modern Architecture: The area's history is visible in its architecture, which means visitors might navigate around or through buildings with varying facades, from old stone and brick to modern glass and steel. This can influence the walking experience, with some pathways or entrances involving steps, ramps, or uneven surfaces.

Streetscape Elements: Expect elements like curbs, crosswalks, and traffic islands that are integral to urban navigation. Street furniture, including lampposts, signage, and bike racks, adds to the navigational landscape but also contributes to a more pedestrian-friendly environment.

Green Spaces: Even in an urban setting, there might be small parks or green areas interspersed, offering grassy or mulched paths, trees, and perhaps flower beds. These spaces provide a softer, more natural terrain amidst the cityscape, ideal for picnics or a respite from concrete.

Accessibility: Efforts to make downtown areas like Rochester Square accessible mean there are likely curb cuts, ramps, and accessible pedestrian signals. However, given the historical nature of some buildings, some areas might be less accessible, requiring alternative routes.

Seasonal Adjustments: Winter in Rochester can bring snow, turning sidewalks into pathways that might be cleared but still require caution due to ice or slush. Conversely, summer might see more outdoor seating or temporary structures for festivals, slightly altering the usual urban terrain.

The terrain of Rochester Square offers a quintessential urban experience, blending historical charm with modern urban planning, providing a walkable, vibrant environment for exploration, shopping, dining, and cultural activities.

Ryan's Notes:

We went to the square kinda by accident, we were coming from Ellison Park. We ended up in downtown Rochester hungry, so we found a parking spot (which wasn't easy) near a barbeque restaurant and bar. Their signature dishes were designed from Tennessee barbeque which isn't spicy but the best barbeque Jamie ever had and I agreed I ate my entire plate which was a lot of food. Once we had lunch we walked outside next to a beautiful waterfall which had tree limbs caught on the aqueducts.

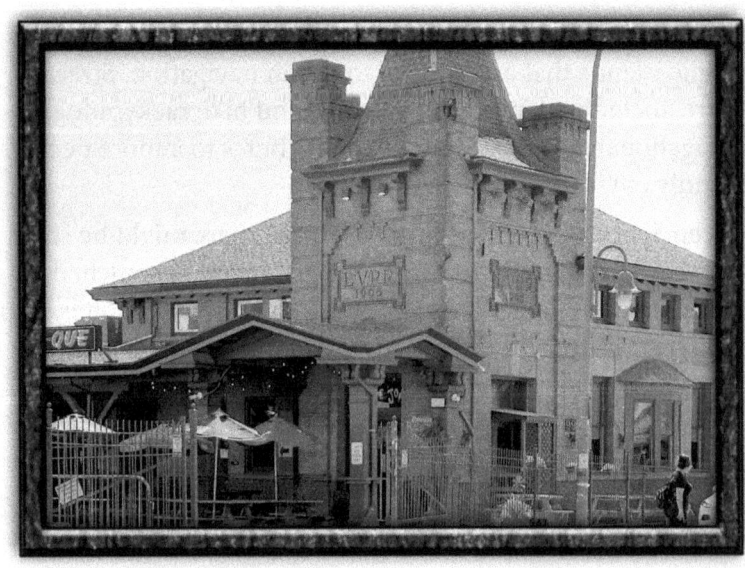

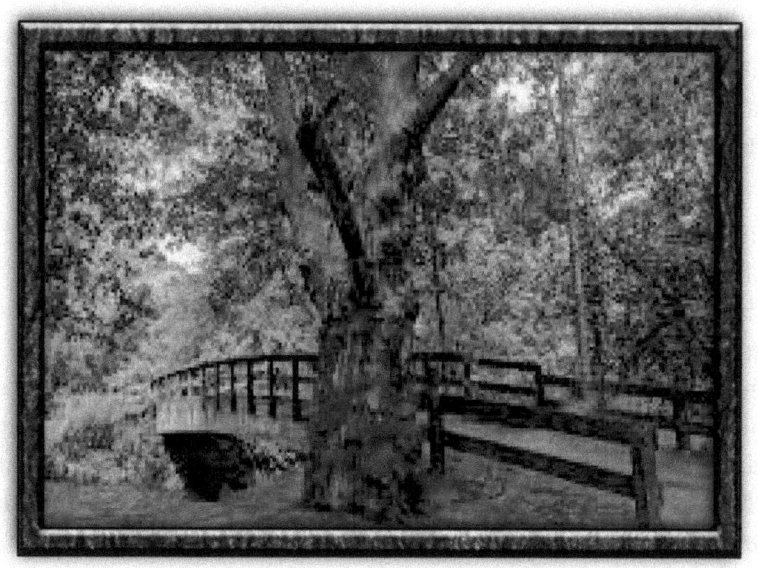

Ellison Park

Location

Ellison Park is located in the town of Penfield, within Monroe County, in Western New York.

The park is situated just east of Rochester, off Blossom Road, making it easily accessible for both city residents and those from surrounding areas. Its proximity to Route 590 and its position along the Irondequoit Creek add to its appeal as a recreational destination. Ellison Park is part of the Monroe County Parks system, offering a blend of urban convenience with natural beauty, set within the scenic landscape of Western New York.

History

Ellison Park's history is a tale of philanthropy, community, and the enduring beauty of nature. Established in December 1926, it became the first official park in the Monroe County Parks system through a generous donation by Mr. and Mrs. Frank T. Ellison. This

200-acre gift was in memory of Frank's father, Nathaniel B. Ellison, showcasing a commitment to providing public access to nature's beauty. Frank T. Ellison, a prominent figure in Rochester's real estate and agriculture sectors, saw the potential in this land to serve as a recreational haven for the growing community.

From the outset, Ellison Park was designed to be a retreat from urban life, with the serene Irondequoit Creek at its heart. The park's early development included the creation of trails, shelters, and sports facilities like baseball and tennis courts, catering to the leisure activities of the time. Its landscape also holds historical significance; the area was once known as Indian Landing, a portage route used by the Seneca Nation, embedding the park with cultural and historical depth. The presence of Fort Schuyler, a replica of an early colonial trading post, further ties the park to the region's past interactions between Native Americans and European settlers.

Over the decades, Ellison Park has not only grown in size, now encompassing 447 acres, but has also evolved in its offerings. The park's expansion involved careful consideration for conservation, ensuring that while new amenities like a disc golf course, an off-leash dog park, and modern playgrounds were added, the natural beauty and ecological integrity of the area were preserved. This balance reflects a broader commitment by Monroe County to maintain public spaces that nurture both community life and environmental stewardship.

Ellison Park has become more than a place for outdoor activities; it's a venue for community events, educational programs, and a spot where countless memories have been made across generations. Its history is intertwined with the story of Monroe County's dedication to providing accessible natural spaces that enhance the quality of life, making Ellison Park a cherished jewel in Western New York's crown of public lands.

Terrain

Visitors to Ellison Park will experience a terrain that blends natural beauty with recreational facilities, offering a diverse landscape for exploration:

Wooded Trails: Much of Ellison Park is forested, with trails that meander through mature woodlands. These paths can range from wide, well-maintained routes suitable for all ages to narrower, more rustic trails that provide a deeper sense of wilderness. The ground here is often covered with leaves, pine needles, or roots, offering a soft, natural walking surface.

Creek Side: Irondequoit Creek runs through the park, providing a scenic backdrop with its banks offering both flat areas for picnicking or fishing and more rugged sections for those looking to explore. The terrain near the creek includes gravel paths, grassy spots, and occasionally rocky or muddy areas depending on recent weather conditions.

Open Fields: There are clearings and open fields within the park, ideal for sports, picnicking, or simply enjoying the sun. These areas are generally flat and grassy, contrasting with the wooded sections and providing space for activities or relaxation.

Recreational Facilities: The park hosts various amenities like tennis courts, a disc golf course, and playgrounds, where the terrain shifts to more structured surfaces like asphalt, concrete, or artificial turf. These areas are designed for specific sports or play, offering a different walking experience compared to the natural trails.

Elevation Changes: Though not extreme, Ellison Park features gentle hills and slopes, particularly around the sledding areas or where trails ascend or descend through the woods. These changes add a bit of challenge to hikes and offer varied vantage points of the park's landscapes.

Seasonal Variations: The terrain at Ellison Park changes with the seasons. Fall brings colorful leaf cover that can make paths slippery, winter might see snow blanketing the trails, altering the walking experience, and spring and summer offer lush vegetation and the sound of the creek at its fullest.

Accessibility: Efforts have been made to ensure some parts of the park are accessible, with paved paths in certain areas to accommodate wheelchairs or strollers. However, the more natural sections of the park might be less accessible due to their ruggedness.

The terrain at Ellison Park invites visitors into a world where urban life fades into the background, replaced by the tranquility of nature, the rush of water, and the joy of outdoor recreation, all within a stone's throw of Rochester.

Ryan's Notes:

Originally we were supposed to go to another park but it ended up to be a YMCA camp so we weren't allowed to be there, so we stopped at a store and asked if there was another park around. They gave us directions and off we went. We drove for a while and found the park. The park lot was huge and Jamie was unsure this was the park until she saw the sign. We got out of the car and off I went, Jamie walks too slow for me plus she likes to take a lot of pictures. I asked do you want to put a leash on me? Because there are a lot of animals she said no my phone is my leash. I said ok! There was an orchard from a neighboring school that had planted a variety of fruits along the paths of one area of the parks. There was also a creek with a wooden bridge to walk over with hills on the one side and the creek on the other. As you walk on the paths some parts of the hill are cleared out with what looks like a maze of flowers. Any age would love to come and spend a day here, have a picnic and just enjoy this place.

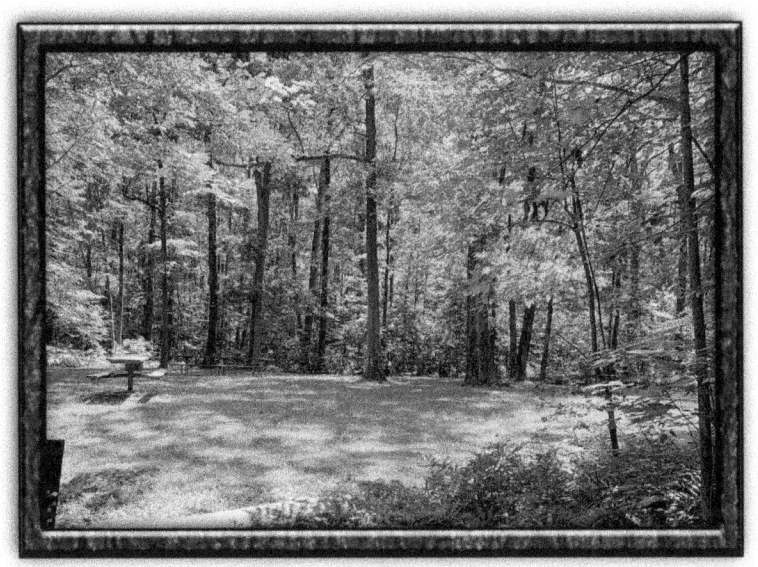

Finger Lakes National Forest

Location

Finger Lakes National Forest is located in the heart of the Finger Lakes region, spanning parts of Schuyler and Seneca Counties in Western New York.

This national forest lies between Seneca Lake and Cayuga Lake, two of the most prominent Finger Lakes, making it easily accessible from various towns in the region, including Ithaca to the south and Watkins Glen to the west. It's roughly 40 miles southwest of Syracuse, providing a convenient natural retreat for those exploring Western New York or the broader Finger Lakes area. The setting of the forest on a ridge between the lakes offers unique landscapes and panoramic views, making it a gem for those seeking natural beauty in the region.

History

The history of Finger Lakes National Forest is a rich tapestry woven from centuries of land use, cultural heritage, and conservation efforts. Before European settlers set foot in the area, it was the homeland of the Iroquois Confederacy, specifically the Seneca and Cayuga Nations, who utilized the land for hunting and gathering, deeply connected to the natural resources that the region, including the lakes Seneca and Cayuga, provided.

The arrival of European settlers, particularly following the Sullivan-Clinton Campaign during the American Revolution, marked a significant shift. This campaign led to the redistribution of land, transforming what was once Native American territory into "military lots" given to soldiers as compensation. This began the transition from a landscape shaped by indigenous practices to one dominated by European-style agriculture, which over time, led to soil depletion and the eventual abandonment of many farms by the early 20th century.

As these farms were left behind, the landscape was dotted with stone walls, old orchards, and the remnants of settlements, telling tales of a once-bustling agricultural community now in decline. The U.S. Soil Conservation Service stepped in during the 1930s, acquiring these lands to combat erosion and restore soil health, marking the beginning of the area's journey towards conservation.

In 1954, the land was handed over to the U.S. Forest Service, and by 1982, it was officially recognized as part of the National Forest System, initially under the name Hector Ranger District, Green Mountain National Forest. It was later renamed Finger Lakes National Forest in 1985, reflecting its unique identity and the shift towards a more holistic approach to land management that included timber production, wildlife conservation, grazing, and recreation.

Today, the forest stands as a testament to the evolution of land use, from indigenous stewardship to agricultural exploitation, and now to conservation and public enjoyment. The historical elements, like old farm structures, are preserved where possible, offering visitors a glimpse into the past while also serving as educational points about the land's history. This national forest not only preserves the natural beauty of the Finger Lakes region but also honors the cultural legacy of those who have lived on and shaped this land over centuries.

Terrain

Visitors to Finger Lakes National Forest will find themselves navigating a terrain that reflects both its natural beauty and its agricultural past:

Rolling Hills and Valleys: The forest is characterized by its gently rolling hills and valleys, offering scenic vistas across the Finger Lakes region. This topography provides for both easy walks and more challenging hikes, with paths that rise and fall with the landscape.

Forest Trails: Much of the forest is covered by deciduous and coniferous trees, with trails weaving through these woods. The ground underfoot varies from soft, leafy paths to more rugged sections with roots and rocks, providing a quintessential hiking experience. Some trails are wide and well-maintained, suitable for families or less experienced hikers, while others offer a more adventurous, less trodden feel.

Open Meadows and Pastures: There are significant areas of open land, remnants of the forest's agricultural history, now managed for wildlife and recreation. These meadows offer flat, grassy areas ideal for picnicking, bird watching, or simply enjoying the wide-open spaces with panoramic views.

Historical Structures: The remnants of old farmsteads, including stone walls and foundations, add a unique dimension to the terrain. These structures can sometimes intersect with trails, offering both navigational landmarks and historical context.

Water Features: While not directly on the lakes, the forest includes smaller water bodies like streams and seasonal wetlands. These areas can introduce wetter, possibly muddy sections to the trails, enhancing the diversity of the hiking experience with the soothing sounds and sights of water.

Seasonal Variations: The terrain changes with the seasons. Autumn transforms the forest into a palette of colors, making for spectacular hikes. Winter might cover the trails in snow, offering opportunities for cross-country skiing or snowshoeing, though this can also mean some paths become less accessible. Spring and summer bring lush vegetation, with wildflowers in the meadows and a vibrant forest canopy.

Accessibility: While much of the forest offers natural, sometimes rugged terrain, there are efforts to provide some accessible paths or viewpoints for those with mobility constraints, though the more remote or steep sections remain challenging.

This diversity in terrain at Finger Lakes National Forest not only caters to various levels of outdoor enthusiasts but also encapsulates the area's history, from its agricultural past to its current conservation ethos, providing a rich, multifaceted experience for all who visit.

Ryan's Notes:

This was our third park on our adventure at Watkins Glen. Jamie parked on the flat surface which they use as a parking lot. We got out and started walking straight up the hill. We ended up walking the entire park while the car was on the other side of the park and we walked down the road to get back to the car. It was a long day. In the park itself you can either walk or drive through there is a paved driveway. On our way back we stopped in someone's driveway and took pictures of the lake.

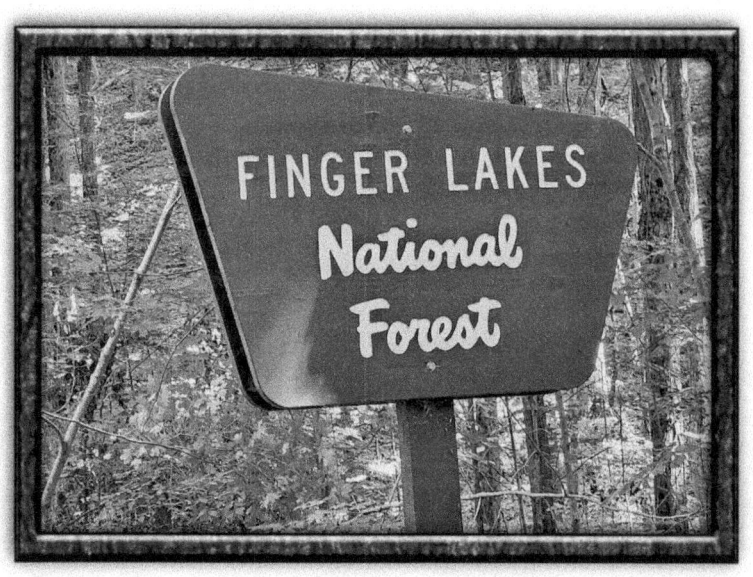

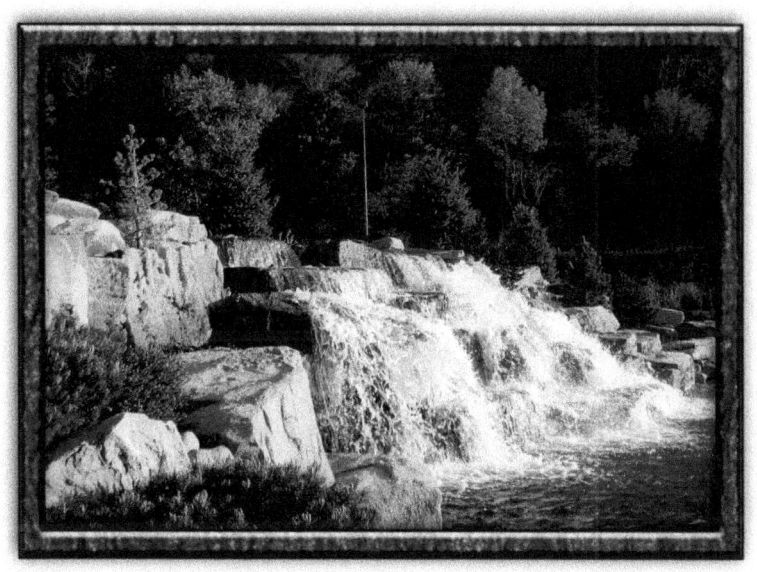

Green Park

Location (This is a place we have yet to see but plan to do when possible)

Green Park is situated in the city of Salamanca, which lies within Cattaraugus County in the southwestern part of New York State.

Salamanca is nestled along the Allegheny River and is part of the Allegany Indian Reservation of the Seneca Nation. Green Park is within the city limits, making it easily accessible for both residents and visitors. The city is approximately 60 miles south of Buffalo and about 80 miles southeast of Niagara Falls, placing it in a region known for its natural beauty, with Allegany State Park nearby. This location makes Green Park a convenient spot for outdoor activities, surrounded by the scenic landscapes of Western New York.

History

The history of Green Park in Salamanca is closely tied to the city's own narrative, shaped by its unique position on the Seneca Nation's Allegany Indian Reservation and its development alongside the railroad industry.

Salamanca was named after José de Salamanca y Mayol, a Spanish noble who invested heavily in the Atlantic and Great Western Railroad, which played a significant role in the town's early growth. The area where Green Park now stands was part of the Seneca Territory long before European settlers arrived, with the Seneca being one of the six nations of the Iroquois Confederacy.

In the late 19th and early 20th centuries, Salamanca became a bustling railroad hub, leading to rapid industrial and population growth. As the city expanded, the need for public spaces became apparent. Green Park, although not extensively documented in historical records, likely emerged from this period as a communal area where residents could gather, a common feature in towns experiencing industrial boom.

The park would have served as a place for community events, relaxation, and recreation, providing a green oasis in what was otherwise a growing industrial landscape. Over the years, as railroads declined and other industries like forestry and tourism took precedence, Green Park has remained a fixture in the community, symbolizing the town's resilience and commitment to maintaining quality of life amidst economic shifts.

The exact timeline of Green Park's establishment isn't well-documented, but it reflects the broader story of Salamanca's adaptation over time - from a railroad town to a community that values its natural and cultural heritage. Today, Green Park stands as a testament to the city's history, offering a space where the past and present of Salamanca converge, with events like community gatherings, picnics, and local celebrations often taking place there.

This park, much like Salamanca itself, embodies the spirit of coexistence between the Seneca Nation and the broader community, highlighting the cultural and historical layers of this unique part of Western New York.

Terrain

Visitors to Green Park in Salamanca will find the terrain to be quite accommodating for a variety of activities, reflecting the park's role as a community gathering space:

Flat and Accessible: The park's primary feature is its level ground, making it easily navigable for people of all ages and abilities. The surface is typically grass or well-trodden earth, suitable for walking, picnicking, or playing games.

Open Spaces: Green Park offers expansive open areas, ideal for sports, community events, or just relaxing on the grass. These areas are relatively flat, providing a simple, enjoyable environment without the need for rugged exploration.

Tree Cover: Mature trees dot the park, offering shade and a touch of natural beauty. These trees not only enhance the park's aesthetics but also create cooler, more comfortable spots for visitors during warmer months.

Walking Paths: While not necessarily a park known for extensive trails, there are likely paths or walkways that crisscross the park, used for leisurely strolls or as connectors between different activity zones. These paths would be straightforward, possibly paved or gravel, ensuring ease of movement.

River Proximity: Although not directly on the Allegheny River, the park's location in Salamanca means it's not far from riverfront areas. This proximity might invite visitors to extend their visit by exploring nearby riverbanks, which would introduce a slight change in terrain with perhaps some gentle slopes or grassy areas leading down to the water.

Seasonal Changes: The terrain at Green Park changes with the seasons, from green and lush in summer to potentially snow-covered in winter, offering different experiences throughout the year. In autumn, the park would be adorned with fallen leaves, while spring might bring the freshness of new growth.

Recreational Facilities: Depending on the amenities provided, there might be playgrounds or sports facilities with surfaces of rubber, asphalt, or other materials tailored for specific activities, adding variety to the park's otherwise flat landscape.

Overall, Green Park provides a straightforward, accessible terrain that's perfect for community gatherings, casual sports, or a quiet day in nature. It's designed to be inclusive, allowing everyone in the community to enjoy the outdoors with minimal challenges from the landscape itself.

Ryan's Notes:

We are looking forward to this and many other adventures this year and the years to come.

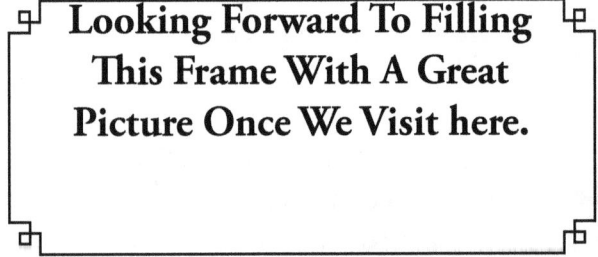

www.ingramcontent.com/pod-product-compliance
Lightning Source LLC
Chambersburg PA
CBHW060851050426
42453CB00008B/941